# I AM YOUR BOOK

## A POETIC JOURNEY THROUGH CFS/ME/FIBROMYALGIA

## Charlotte Jones

**BALBOA.**
PRESS
A DIVISION OF HAY HOUSE

Balboa Press books may be ordered through booksellers or by contacting:

Balboa Press
A Division of Hay House
1663 Liberty Drive
Bloomington, IN 47403
www.balboapress.com
1 (877) 407-4847

Print information available on the last page.

ISBN: 978-1-9822-0685-7 (sc)
ISBN: 978-1-9822-0687-1 (hc)
ISBN: 978-1-9822-0686-4 (e)

Library of Congress Control Number: 2018907353

Balboa Press rev. date: 07/10/2019

For Dom

My Hubby
My Hero
My light when all was dark

x

# CONTENTS

# HELLO FROM YOUR BOOK

# HELLO FROM YOUR BOOK

Welcome to your book,

Whether you have CFS/ME/Fibromyalgia, know someone with it, treat people with it, or know nothing about it, I am the book for you.

For those of you with CFS/ME/Fibromyalgia; I'm not here to give you a quick fix cure. I'm just here to share the rhythm of this journey to let you know that you are not alone.

Inside me you will find something to befriend you on your lonely days, to hold your hand on your tough days, to motivate you on your give-up days, to provide a shoulder on your sad days, to high-five you on your happy days and to be there for you on your everydays.

For those of you who don't have CFS/ME/Fibromyalgia; by sharing this story I hope to raise awareness of the illness and provide you with an insight into the potential life of those who do.

Whatever your reason for being here with me now, I am your book. I do not adhere to normal book rules. You can do with me as you please. You can read me from front to back to follow the rollercoaster of emotions, or you can flick to a random page. You can skip right to the end or read the same page over and over. *You can get a little context to each poem (see 'Setting the Scene' at the back of the book) or you can let the poems tell their own story. You can highlight me. Underline me. Doodle on me. Rhyme on me. Find the poem that catches your soul, rip it out and stick it on your wall or read it to a loved one to show them how you feel. Don't hold on to me for posterity purposes. I'm here to help you in the present moment. I'm here for you right now. Enjoy!*

*Love from*
    *Your Book x*

# WHAT'S IN A NAME?

# WHAT'S IN A NAME?

## CFS/ME/Fibromyalgia

It is generally accepted that CFS (Chronic Fatigue Syndrome) and ME (Myalgic Encephalomyelitis) are the same thing. They are often referred to as CFS/ME. There is however a lot of debate in the medical world around where Fibromyalgia fits into this.

Are CFS/ME and Fibromyalgia the same thing just with an emphasis on different symptoms; CFS/ME with an emphasis on fatigue and Fibromyalgia with an emphasis on pain? Are they similar and from the same family of illness but with some very specific differences between the two? Or are they completely different, with nothing in common but a few symptoms?

I am in no way qualified to enter into this debate so shall remain firmly out of it. There is a lot of research looking into both CFS/ME and Fibromyalgia at the moment so I hope this will soon shed some light on the situation.

In the meantime, what I can talk about is my own experience; I was primarily diagnosed with CFS/ME, but as I was also suffering from extreme debilitating pain all over my body, I ended up with a diagnosis of CFS/ME and Fibromyalgia.

For the sake of ease, I used to just refer to it as CFS. As I have used this term throughout all of my poems I shall continue to use the term CFS to encompass CFS/ME and Fibromyalgia throughout the rest of the book.

For those of you who have been diagnosed with Fibromyalgia, please don't feel this in any way means that this book isn't for you. I am your book too.

# THE STORY
# BEHIND THE BOOK

# THE STORY BEHIND THE BOOK

When I was five years old my Grannie took me to see some giant cows at a neighbouring farm. Looking back, I don't suppose they were any bigger than normal cows, I'd just never been that close before. It was such an amazing day that I could hardly contain my excitement and I had words repeating rhythmically in my head. When we arrived back at my Grandparent's cottage I knew I had to get these words out of my head. I ran into my room, grabbed a pen and let the words spill out onto the page...

> *I went to see some cows today.*
> *Some white, some brown, some black.*

That was it. So simple. I felt so much better once the words were out on paper! I ran into the kitchen to show my Gran. "Look Grannie, look what I've written!". My Gran took the paper from me and read the words out loud. I remember her exact response; "Ooo that's lovely dear, why don't we write another line and make it into a poem!?". Excited at the thought, I sat down next to my Grannie and we hashed out another line turning it into my first ever poem:

> *I went to see some cows today*
> *Some white, some brown, some black*
> *They stared at me with great big eyes*
> *I stood and stared them back!*

I have taken pen to paper with poetry often since that day but always just presumed I was a sporadic poet dipping in and out when I fancied it. The last few years however have highlighted a method in my madness. It turns out that poetry is my coping mechanism for dealing with extremes in life. A way of setting emotions free. When I am experiencing extreme highs or lows, my mind repeats a line of poetry over and over, again and again, until I grab a pen and let it loose. The rest of the poem then spills out onto the page releasing whatever extreme emotion I am experiencing. Looking back at my life this now explains my random relationship with poetry and how this book came into being.

I had CFS for three years and CFS is a world of extremes; highs and lows, hopes and disappointments, pain and joy, courage and despair. At the end of my journey I had written hundreds of poems, each one a little window into my soul. The poems I have selected for this book will take you along with me through the wilderness of my journey. They are raw, personal and explicit, as they were only ever intended to be a private release for myself. They have not been edited or amended since their original conception, as to soften them for poetry's sake would somehow compromise the spirit in which they were written.

I was at first reluctant to publish these poems as they are essentially a diary of the toughest times of my life. Looking back now, thankfully free from the daily struggles of CFS, I can see a bigger picture. One where these poems can help others. Not just those suffering from CFS, but also their loved ones, their Doctors, and researchers.

I also hope that this book can serve to raise awareness of CFS in general. Despite the fact that millions of people suffer from CFS around the globe, it is an illness which is rarely spoken about and is gravely misunderstood. Due to the nature of the illness it is often met with disbelief and many think you should just be able to "get out of bed". I don't blame these people; maybe I would have thought the same if I were them. What this means though is that many people with CFS can spend a lot of their very precious energy trying to prove to people in their life that they are really ill, whilst simultaneously trying to prove that they are doing everything in their power to get better. This can result in a hopeless struggle that only serves to make the symptoms of CFS more severe.

I am hoping that by raising awareness of CFS and its symptoms, people will be more accepting of the illness and begin to understand not only what people with CFS go through on a daily basis, but also what they can do to help them. This will mean that CFS sufferers will be able to conserve their limited energy for healing and relax into the healing state their body needs to recover.

Due to the lack of understanding around CFS, it can be a very lonely journey. So I hope that if you do have CFS these poems will make you feel understood, and maybe even make you smile. I'm not trying to scare you with images of my struggle. I'm not even trying to motivate you to a recovery (although I hope my happy ending gives you hope and spurs you on towards yours!). What I am hoping to do with this book is share the rhythm of my journey to let you know that you are not alone.

For those of you who know people or are treating people with CFS, I hope that this book gives you a good insight into how they may be feeling day-to-day. I often found it hard to find the words to explain to my husband exactly what I was going through. Luckily on my darkest days when I needed him most my poems would flow freely, giving me a way of sharing my journey with him. It was my husband who first encouraged me to share my poems with the world in the hope that others could benefit from them in the same way that we did.

Whatever your reason for reading this book, I hope that you enjoy these little windows into my soul as together we travel the ups and downs of the rollercoaster journey that is CFS.

# INTRODUCTION

# INTRODUCTION

## What is CFS?

CFS (Chronic Fatigue Syndrome) is a long-term debilitating illness which causes extreme fatigue that can't be fixed with sleep or rest. Other symptoms include muscle pain, brain fog and sleeping difficulties (too much, too little or inadequate quality).

If you read that bit again it doesn't seem that bad does it? Fatigue, pain, and trouble sleeping. Surely everyone feels like this after a stressful day at work or an extensive session down the gym?... Thus begins the story of how CFS is one of the most misunderstood illnesses we have today.

One of the first reasons for this misunderstanding is that our vocabulary doesn't have words to suitably describe what CFS sufferers go through. The closest words we have are 'exhaustion' or 'fatigue', and once someone hears these words they just presume that you are 'tired'.

**Comparing CFS to tiredness is like comparing the Antarctic to an everyday ice cube.**

I spent three years with CFS, throughout which I was predominantly bed bound, literally unable to move and in absolute agony. Vocab such as 'tired' or 'muscle pain' didn't even scratch the surface of how I was feeling.

Another reason is that people with CFS can often look absolutely fine, so it is hard for others to see that they are even ill. The nature of the illness also means that people can often do something one day that they are physically incapable of doing the next day, so this again adds to the misconceptions and disbelief around the illness.

CFS is a world of unknowns. There is currently a lot of research going on around the globe looking into CFS; What is it? How do we get it? Why do we get it? How can we recover? For now, there are no concrete answers to any of these questions, so we just have to go on the information we have.

There are many predisposing factors that lead up to someone getting CFS and then there is usually a trigger that is the final straw that sets off the symptoms. This trigger causes the body to crash, and because the body then becomes incapable of regenerating energy, it is unable to repair itself.

Everybody's experience of CFS is different and the severity of symptoms can vary from person to person. Some can carry on with a semi-normal life just at a slower pace. Others, like myself, are bed-bound for years. A lucky few recover within a few months, others a few years and some live with it their entire lives.

There are currently no lab tests to show if you have CFS, so diagnosis is by way of elimination. As the symptoms of CFS are common to so many other illnesses, some people have to wait months or even years before ruling everything else out and getting a diagnosis.

This delay can cause a lot of stress and anxiety which unfortunately does not disappear upon diagnosis. The many unknowns of CFS means it can be hard for people to understand what is happening to them, what they need to do to recover, or how to explain it to family/friends/employers. One of the requirements for a recovery is to be in a relaxed stress-free state of healing which allows the body to repair, so this stress and anxiety can actually serve to make the situation worse and spiral a person deeper into the grasps of CFS.

Two years into my journey I went to a private CFS clinic in London called the Optimum Health Clinic. It was at this point that I finally started to get some answers to my many questions surrounding CFS. The clinic was able to help me understand more about why I had CFS, what was going on inside my body and what steps I could take to recover.

I learnt that there are many systems in the body that can malfunction simultaneously when you have CFS; your energy system, digestive system and immune system, to name a few. It was learning about Mitochondrial Malfunction and the Maladaptive Stress Response that really helped me get my head around what was happening to me. These are very simplified explanations:

**'Mitochondrial Malfunction'** - the energy in your cells is not recycling properly so you only have a very small percentage of energy compared to healthy people.

**'Maladaptive Stress Response'** – your body becomes so weak and is put under so much pressure that it starts to perceive everything as a threat to its survival. Your body therefore kicks in its inbuilt response to danger (fight, flight or freeze) so often that it actually becomes normalised. Whilst in this stress response of fight, flight or freeze, your body shuts down non-essential activities (like digestion and immunity) so it can divert the energy to bodily functions that help you quickly 'get out of danger'. This is great for short term threats like jumping out of the way of a bus, yet crippling after long term constant use.

Knowing more about what was going on inside my body helped me relax more into my recovery journey. I also felt a lot less pressure when trying to explain to people what was wrong with me. The knowledge and evidence added gravitas to my explanation and helped me feel more understood and less judged.

## Is There a Cure to CFS?

There are some medical professionals who will tell you that there is no cure to CFS and that you can only learn to manage your symptoms. If your definition of a cure is a quick-fix pill or procedure, then this could be considered true. There are however many, many people (such as myself) who have fully recovered from CFS who are testament to there being a cure.

The problem is that, as every case of CFS is different, there is no one-size-fits-all cure. There are often multiple systems in the body malfunctioning at the same time, the illness itself has different stages which are receptive to different treatments, and each person reacts differently to any attempts at recovery. This can often make recovery extremely complicated and mean that each person has to find their own unique path back to health.

## My Reality of CFS

So what is it actually like to live with CFS?

Every case is different, but here is what my day to day life was like with CFS:

In the preliminary stage (the Crash stage) I slept for 20 hours a day and felt like I hadn't slept a wink. It was as if my body had completely shut down on me. It felt like I was the Duracell bunny and someone had taken out my batteries. I was in so much pain it felt like my bones were being crushed by The Hulk and my skin had been set on fire. It felt like a ten-tonne truck was pinning me down to the bed so I couldn't move. When I could get out of bed, I was so weak my legs couldn't hold my body up for more than a few seconds, my neck couldn't hold my head up without support and my arms couldn't hold my hands up long enough to do basic things like eat with a knife and fork or brush my teeth. I would often have to crawl to the bathroom and need to be carried up the stairs. My head felt like it was full of cotton wool making it impossible to think and everything felt numb.

My husband describes my worst times as 'The Ghost-Times'. I would be lying in bed or sitting on the sofa chatting to him and my body would just shut down. I would go completely still, my eyes would glaze over and all of the blood would drain from my face and limbs making me look almost translucent. He admits to thinking I was dead the first time it happened, but it was just my body's way of shutting down to conserve energy. This happened regularly throughout my Crash stage, my body was so weak that even lying in bed and having a conversation used up too much energy.

In the second stage (the Tired and Wired stage) it was like I was being ripped from the quiet, numb little cocoon I'd been living in during the previous stage. It was such a shock to the senses that my body felt constantly under attack and saw everything as a threat. So despite the fact that the exhaustion from the previous stage was still present, I was now unable to sleep as my whole body felt like it was pulsing with adrenaline to keep me alive from these perceived threats. As the cotton wool cloud lifted from over my head, certain noises, lights and even smells were too much and brought on panic attacks. I was therefore left with crippling anxiety. I had PTSD (Post-Traumatic Stress Disorder) on top of this, with flashbacks to my close calls in hospital, which was a particularly harrowing part of my journey.

During this second stage I was able to get out of bed some days, but my physical abilities were very limited. My pain actually became worse, which I wouldn't have thought possible. My emotions flicked between hope on my good days and pure disappointment and despair on my bad days.

You will hear more about the daily struggles of living with CFS in my poems. Another reoccurring theme you will read about is loneliness:

**Regardless of how many loved ones surround you and support you, you are lonely. No one in the world can really understand what you're going through unless they've been there themselves and, as every journey is different, maybe not even then.**

CFS, no matter what your symptoms, can be a very lonely illness. Cripplingly lonely. I spent most of my journey feeling like no one really knew what it was, no one could really help me, and that lots of people didn't even believe me. I felt alone, in pain, alienated from my former life and desperate to get better without a clue where to start. It wasn't until I released this urgent desperation to get better and relaxed enough to put my body into a healing state that I could even begin my recovery journey. Here is my story...

# MY STORY

# MY STORY

The poems in this book were written over a three-year period in my early 30's when I was suffering with CFS. This was actually the second time that I'd had CFS, the first was in my early 20's. I now believe that CFS was in my life for a reason. It was my body's way of trying to communicate with me and tell me that something wasn't quite right. Both times I had felt *lost*, and it was CFS that had found me.

Having CFS forced me to stop and reassess life. During my first encounter with CFS I learnt lessons that helped me lead a happier, healthier life that was truer to myself. Somewhere along the way I forgot these lessons and, after a few years, fell back into living my life for others and ended up back where I started. Lost.

Once again, it was CFS who found me and once again, it had lessons to teach me. Harder lessons this time round. Lessons that involved years of agony, despair and soul searching. Lessons that I wouldn't swap for the world, because they led me to where I am right now. CFS forced me to listen, forced me to get to know myself, forced me to let love in and forced me to learn how to bring light into my own world.

I am grateful for all that CFS taught me and wish that I could use all that I have learnt to wave a magic wand and make anyone suffering with CFS instantly better. Unfortunately though, this is not how CFS works. CFS is not something that someone can rescue you from. You have to be your own hero, your own saviour. You have to fight in order to learn to let go, you have to be in pain in order to learn to listen to your body, you have to be exhausted in order to stop long enough to reassess life. Only you can learn the lessons you need to learn. Only you can be your own hero.

> **"We do not receive wisdom, we must discover it for ourselves, after a journey through the wilderness which no one else can make for us, which no one can spare us, for our wisdom is the point of view from which we come at last to regard the world."**
>
> Marcel Proust

Although I cannot provide you with an instant cure to CFS, I do hope that by sharing my poems, my story and the lessons I have learnt, you will be able to take some short cuts on your own journey towards health.

This is my story....

## CFS: The First Time

I had my first encounter with CFS when I was 22. The years leading up to this were full on, hardworking, fun years. I was an over-achiever, a happy, bouncy, go-getter who had to do her best at everything she turned her hand to and had to always push to do that little bit extra. University alone hadn't felt like enough of a challenge for me so I got a job working as a Buyer for a large international company who sponsored me through my degree. I squeezed a full-time job, a full-time degree and a full on social life into each week. I can honestly say it was a fun, jam packed life. Until one day it wasn't...

I was always such a happy smiley person so at the time didn't think anything was amiss. With hindsight, however, I can see that this was not the case. I loved my job but I never really felt like I was where I was meant to be. I can now see that I always felt like there was something missing, something more that I couldn't quite get to. I would continuously push myself further in hope that this missing link was hiding behind the next achievement. Of course it never was. I was always looking externally for my happiness and self-worth in belief that they could be obtained from grades, jobs, relationships, achievements, experiences and most importantly from the approval of others. I never grasped that happiness came from within.

I liked the people I worked with, I had some great colleagues who are still my close friends to this day and my boss was caring, supportive and a fantastic mentor. He always made sure I was recognised and rewarded for my hard work and he made work a happy place to be. This meant that I liked going to work, and I didn't think I could ask for anything more. So why did I feel so unfulfilled? I loved to learn, so whilst studying for my degree I felt like I had a greater purpose, something to work towards, but once I graduated I felt lost and never really recovered from this feeling. I began to realise that the current path I was on wasn't right for me, but didn't know what to do about it. It was all I had known. One day I was sitting at my desk and the guy next to me was retiring and I remember thinking "I wonder which desk I'll be sitting at when I retire?". I was only 22 at the time and it was quite a sobering thought. I could only see myself following this one same path for the rest of my life and I knew it wasn't my life's purpose. There had to be another way, but I didn't know how to access it.

I believe now that we are all here on earth to follow a certain path and when we're on that path, we feel relaxed, at home and content in our own skin. When we stray from this path we feel like there is always something missing and our body will try to find ways to alter our course. I believe that CFS was my body's way of forcing me to find an alternative path in life.

Living out of line with my soul purpose, alongside the constant pushing and striving in my life, led to a gradual build-up of long-term stresses on the body and mind. My body gave me warning signs in the form of exhaustion, constant headaches and reoccurring throat, ear and chest infections. I pushed through these, only serving to make the situation even worse. I don't blame myself for this, I didn't know any better at the time.

Then one day, at a Christmas Ball of all places, I just crashed. I felt like I was having a heart attack (this pain was suspected to be a symptom of the virus that was my trigger for CFS). So there I was, at a Christmas ball, hiding in the toilet, stripped half naked (as my dress became too tight on my chest), eagerly awaiting my mate to come rescue me with a coat and take me home.

This still didn't stop me though. Come Monday morning I was in work as usual, but I passed out before I even got to my desk. My boss sent me home and that was that. I was in bed for the next year with CFS.

Throughout the year I tried desperately to get better so I could get back to work. After 6 months of being completely bedbound I did attempt a few hours of work here and there. I either worked from home or pushed myself to get into the office for a few hours, but each time I would crash and end up back in bed.

My Doctor introduced me to a fabulous lady who taught me Chi Kung. I instantly took to it and embraced it fully, practicing what little I could every day. It brought me hope as I felt like I finally had something I could physically do each day to work towards my recovery.

After just over a year, I finally accepted that the life I was trying to push myself back into wasn't right for me. This led to a speedy recovery. It's like the sudden change in direction shifted my energy and released me from the shackles of CFS.

My moment of realisation came on my birthday. My Mum came round to take me out for lunch but I was so tired all I wanted to do was sleep. Mum sat down next to me and asked me a question which was one of the most important questions of my life. She said **"What do _YOU_ really want to do with your life? What would make _YOU_ happy?"** ... ... ...

I was absolutely stumped... ... I realised I had never really stopped to ask myself this question. I had lived my entire life doing what I thought I SHOULD do. I was an optimistic happy person so had always found happiness in everything I had done, but is this true happiness if you are living out of line with your inner self? With hindsight I can now see that instead of looking internally to see what would have made *me* genuinely happy, I was looking externally and conforming to expectations of society. Oscar Wilde sums it up beautifully here:

> **"There are moments when one has to choose between living one's own life, fully, entirely, completely – or dragging out some false, shallow, degrading existence that the world in its hypocrisy demands. You have that moment now. Choose. Oh my love, Choose."**
>
> Oscar Wilde

That was my moment. Right there, sitting talking to my Mum on my birthday. The first time I truly asked myself not what I thought I should do but what _I_ truly wanted to do? Who _I_ truly wanted to be? I loved the freedom and genuine happiness that came from asking that question and it opened me up to a new life of health, happiness and freedom.

My answer to the question was simple; I had always wanted to do a ski season. I could hardly walk at the time, let alone ski, so we agreed that I should start with my second option which was to sit on a beach for a few months to recover. With my new-found sense of freedom and my Mum's response of "Go do it Dear!" I resigned the next day and set off for Australia. The 'sitting' never happened as the new challenges and outlook in life shifted my energy enough to help me recover quickly. When I arrived I couldn't even carry my backpack and had to drag it behind me, yet after a few weeks of sunshine and freedom I was fully living: road trips, white water rafting, driving up sand dunes, riding horses down the beach, and swimming with sharks.

I spent the next few years full of health, travelling around the world and doing some exciting 'work' (I'm not sure I can call it work as it always felt more like play). I wanted to experience the world and see what life had to offer. I turned toward my love of photography and worked on a boat in Australia photographing scuba divers on the Great Barrier Reef. I photographed big bands at gigs and music festivals which was tonnes of fun. I photographed premiership football games, and I did loads of portraiture work which I loved. I also did some random short term jobs whilst travelling, just to experience real life where I was living; I served scrumptious food in an Italian restaurant where the owners loved to fatten me up with their delicious Spag Bol. Another time, I went into a pizzeria to get a pizza - they were in a panic because the delivery guy was sick – ten minutes later I left with a name badge, a car that had a giant plastic pizza on the top of it and a stack of pizzas to deliver. I loved this life of freedom and adventure and my health continued to thrive as a result of it.

A few years later I finally did that ski season and I absolutely loved it. I was the first one on the slopes every morning to experience that fresh snow. It was a dream come true.

I met a guy whilst skiing and after the season we moved to settle down in his hometown where I found a nice job working on educational projects in Africa and India. After a few years I started to feel a little lost again, like I wasn't where I was meant to be. Looking back, I can see that I had lost the joy that I had so lovingly discovered over the previous years, and once again I was living life for others and conforming to expectations of society. I began to realise that the relationship I was in, and the life I was living, weren't right for me, but I didn't know what to do about it. I felt 'stuck'. Eventually this began to take its toll on my health and I started to get migraines again for the first time in years. This brings us to the lead up to my second time with CFS in my early 30s, during which time I wrote the poems in this book.

## CFS: The Second Time

I left the relationship I was in and, although I knew this was the right thing to do, it left me with a gaping hole in my life. I felt like I had no direction. I felt completely lost.

To make matters worse, I was living far away from my family and friends and was desperate to get back home, so I took the quickest path possible to make that happen. This path involved working in the same job I was doing all those years ago when I first became ill with CFS, this time at a different company. Even though I knew the job wasn't right for me, I enjoyed it to begin with because I met some fun people and I was happy to be home. Unfortunately, this enjoyment soon wore off. I was exhausted, often working in two to three different countries each week, I didn't have the right people in my team to support me, and the work itself was nothing like in my last role. I was often forced to make business decisions that went against my morals, and I found this soul crushing.

I started to get the warning signs of throat, ear and chest infections again and knew I had to get out of this situation. I found a new job that I thought would be more aligned with my soul, organising a charity project for schools in Africa. My hope was that this shift of energy would help nourish my soul back to health, but unfortunately this wasn't the case, and my health continued to deteriorate. A few months later, I got home from a work trip to Africa and I just crashed. I couldn't move. I felt like someone had taken out my batteries. I knew the symptoms from ten years previous, and my Doctor confirmed - I had CFS.

I couldn't believe I had CFS again! I literally couldn't get out of bed. It was like a ten-tonne truck was sitting on me. It felt ten times worse than before. There was no speedy recovery for me this time around. It was a very long journey to a very new life.

Having already made a full recovery from CFS was both a blessing and a curse. I primarily had a confidence that I would recover quickly as I had already done it once. However, last time I had just fallen into a recovery after a shift of energy and direction. That didn't work this time round, so I was left feeling demoralised and demotivated, aimlessly searching for answers.

Over the next few months I pushed myself to get better so I could return to work but I just seemed to get worse and worse. The pressure I felt to return to work was immense. My health continued to deteriorate and I eventually lost my job. I then lost my house and had to move back in with my parents. I was very fortunate to have my parents there to support me and welcome me home with open arms, and luckily my Dad had just retired so he was able to look after me each day.

I spent most of my time bedbound and was unable to do the most basic tasks such as brush my teeth or wash my hair. I had to drag myself to get to the toilet. I couldn't hold my head up so had to constantly lean it on a chair or bed or wall. I had to eat with plastic knives and forks and drink through a straw as I wasn't strong enough to pick up cutlery and cups. If I tried to walk my legs would just give way and I would end up crawling. I would lie in bed unable to move, unaware of how many days had passed. It was a very sorry existence.

## The White Light

Soon after moving home, my Doctor and I wondered whether something else was going on as well as CFS because I was getting so much worse. I was losing weight fast yet eating at an incredible rate. Day and night. I would wake up in the night and have to eat a full meal just to see me through to the morning. I was treated for parasites but little changed. I had lost all of the colour in my face and my skin was almost translucent. It seemed like I was unable to gain any nutrients from the food I was eating.

A few weeks later I caught the flu and my body was so weak I was unable to fight it properly. I was rushed to hospital and soon lost the ability to breath unassisted. Once they found out I had been poorly since my trip to Africa I was put on the isolation ward all alone. During my stay in the hospital, I nearly lost my life twice, once in the emergency room and another in the isolation ward. These are what I call my 'white light moments'. On both occasions I was in absolute agony and struggling to breathe, then a feeling of peace came over me, the need to breathe disappeared and my pain just vanished, so I remember feeling almost welcoming of the situation. Luckily, on both occasions, someone had been there to save me. Both the fact that I had nearly died, and the fact that I had almost welcomed the feeling, truly haunted me.

They did lots of tests in hospital to try to work out what was wrong with me and found I had a dangerously enlarged spleen and cirrhosis (scarring) of the liver. They said it looked like damage from a tropical disease I must have caught in Africa. They said this could potentially be what was causing all of my symptoms. Once I was strong enough to leave the hospital they sent me to the Hospital for Tropical Disease in London.

## The Hope

The diagnosis of a potential tropical disease actually made me hopeful. Every attempt I had made to recover from CFS had not worked, so maybe this was the answer? Maybe I didn't have CFS again? Maybe the Hospital Doctors were right and I had a tropical disease that could potentially be cured with a quick fix pill or procedure? Or maybe I did have CFS and the tropical disease was my trigger, and so once this was cured, my recovery from CFS would be easier? I was full of hope.

Over the next four months I visited the Hospital for Tropical Disease every week or two whilst they tried to work out what was wrong with me. Getting to the hospital in London in my state was a massive challenge in itself. Looking back, a wheelchair would have been a sensible option, but I refused one at the time because I feared that if I got into one I would never get out of it. Instead my (now) hubby or my Dad would carry me or hold me up whilst I shuffled from home to taxi, to train, to taxi, to hospital.

It was always a gruelling journey and by the time I got home I could barely function. I remember one time in the taxi, I was so exhausted the signals between my brain and my mouth were getting crossed and I was trying to say 'car' but kept saying 'camel'. It sounds quite funny now, but at the time it was really frustrating. I would then just crash in bed for the next few days trying to recover before doing it all over again. I never minded making this journey though, because I always went to the hospital full of hope. I had the UK's top specialist for tropical disease working on my case and he promised he would find out what was wrong with me.

Four months later, the Doctor had to admit defeat as he couldn't find a specific tropical disease that could be causing all of the symptoms. He did find evidence of other viruses that could have been triggers for CFS, but they didn't explain the scarring on the liver. He said that the medical field only knew of a small percentage of the tropical diseases out there, so whatever had caused the scarring on my liver would remain a mystery. The quest for answers stopped as my liver began to heal itself and my spleen returned to normal. If there was a tropical disease, it had now gone, and as I still had all of the symptoms of CFS, I was right back where I started.

For months I had lived with the hope that the Doctor would find a tropical disease that was causing all of my symptoms (or making the CFS worse) and be able to cure it and make me better. I had also lived with the fear that he wouldn't find it quick enough and I would die whilst waiting. I was now split between celebrating the recovery of my liver, and being absolutely gutted to be back with the sole diagnosis of CFS. I felt so hopeless again, so alone, with nowhere to turn for help.

## The Love

During this time, I fell in love. Heart swelling, life changing, soul settling love. I had found my man. He always says I had to be in a coma to let him in, which we laugh about, but I suppose in a way is true. I had known him for years but always thought he was too good for me. He didn't need 'fixing' so what good was I to him? I had tangled my self-worth up in a web of helping others and without that I didn't know who I was. Being so poorly I was unable to run away from my feelings, unable to hide them under activities and so I finally opened up and let him in. I let him love me. Let him help me. Let him be there for me. Something I had not let any other man do. I fell hook, line and sinker.

He brought sunshine into my life and loved me unconditionally, giving me the space and security to discover who I really was inside. We bought a house together, travelled the ups and downs of a life with CFS, and dreamt of getting married and having a little family once I'd recovered.

## The Struggle

By the time I had been discharged from the Hospital for Tropical Disease I'd already had CFS for a whole year. At this point my pain was so excruciating I could barely cope. It felt like my bones were being crushed by The Hulk, my muscles were being ripped to shreds and my skin was on fire. At its worst I would be screaming in agony. Other times, the non-stop bone crushing pressure would leave me lying there silently sobbing, tears streaming down my face. I tried prescription pain meds but they didn't make any difference.

It was too painful to even lie down and I used to dream of floating in a cloud so nothing touched my body. Even the slightest touch felt as heavy as lead and a hug was just unbearable and caused excruciating pain. I couldn't find any clothes that didn't hurt me so I spent most of my time wearing my Dad's extra-large T shirts and some really loose pyjama bottoms so they barely touched me.

The next year was a constant struggle to get better. I was predominantly still bedbound and had very little energy. What energy I did have I spent reading up on CFS and putting into place things that people recommended I do to get better. Some helped a little, some made me worse. I was pushing so hard towards a recovery that it was actually counterproductive, as it put my weak body under more stress. I barely had enough energy and mental capacity to survive each day, so the rollercoaster journey that I went through this year was absolutely soul crushing.

In my search for answers I did find some very magical people who helped me along my way...

## The Help

My Gran recommended I have aromatherapy to help ease my pain, so I went in search of an Aromatherapist. Who knew this one action would change my entire life and open up my world to so many new things.

I found a fantastic holistic healer, close to my home, who practiced aromatherapy. She recalls the day that my husband carried me into her shop, looked her in the eye and pleaded with her to help us. We were desperate for some help to reduce the pain and suffering. Luckily we were guided to the right place.

This wonderful Angel (as she is still referred to in our house) treated me with Aromatherapy, Reflexology, Crystal Therapy and Angelic Reiki. Along the way she taught me all about energy. She introduced me to holistic medicines and alternative perspectives on healing. She helped me recognise the support and love of the universe and understand the power that we all hold within us to heal and repair ourselves. She opened my eyes to a new universe full of love, light and opportunity. I will forever be grateful for her and all that she has taught me. The day I walked into her shop was a massive turning point, not just in my healing journey, but also in my life.

I then found a Nutritionist to revamp my diet to reduce any stresses on the body. I quit sugar, caffeine, gluten and dairy and she found me new alternatives to help boost my energy. She also found supplements that helped increase my energy and reduce my pain a little, which made daily life more bearable.

*(If you have CFS, please don't self-medicate any supplements. I had many tests to find out what my body needed before finding the right supplements for me. Please find a qualified nutritionist who specialises in CFS to find out exactly what you need).*

I was extremely lucky to have a very supportive Doctor throughout my time with CFS. He always went above and beyond and found ways to help guide me down my recovery path. He gave me books to read that opened my eyes to more mindful ways of living. On his recommendation I followed Jon Kabat-Zinn's amazing MBSR (Mindfulness-based stress reduction) program which uses techniques like meditation to help you cope better with pain and illness. He also gave me exercises to do that helped me bring much needed snippets of joy into my life. I had been finding it very difficult to think of anything positive because I was so exhausted and constantly in pain, so these exercises really helped me shift my perspective.

As I started to see some gradual improvements in my health, I was able to get out of bed some days and get around the house. I was able to hold my head up without support and could walk a few steps unaided which really opened up my life. My lovely hubby-to-be organised some fun days out for us that didn't involve much physical activity. My family were also really fab at taking me places and organising it so I didn't have to walk anywhere, they always did it as if it was completely normal, which I really appreciated.

## The Re-Runs

Now that my body had gained a little more strength, my brain fog was able to lift a little and my mind started to wake up. It felt like I was being ripped out of a numb little cocoon and my senses went into overdrive. I couldn't cope with certain noises like the TV or music or the tumble dryer or too many people talking at once. I also became a little sensitive to light and smell, but it was the noises that literally floored me.

As my mind woke up even more, I started to remember the details from my time in hospital. When I had come out of hospital I had been unable to process what had happened to me in my 'white light moments'. My whole perception of a secure happy life had literally been turned upside down. I couldn't make sense of all the questions running through my head; How could life be taken from you so easily? The process of letting go was so peaceful, and with it my pain and the constant struggle to breathe disappeared, but even so, how could I have even contemplated letting go!? How was it even possible to not be breathing yet still be alive enough to register you weren't breathing? What was the white light? What if I hadn't gone to hospital when I did? What if the Doctor didn't walk in when he did? What? Why? How?... the questions went on and on and on...

Unable to process all of these questions my brain had just literally shut down and stored the memories away so they didn't haunt me. With my mind not working properly, I hadn't even realised this had happened. I had presumed I was experiencing a bit of brain fog which is a common symptom of CFS, but it was more than that. My mind had been blanking out memories to protect me from having to process it all whilst I was so weak. I had remembered being in hospital but not any of the specifics. Then all this time later, just as I started to see some improvements in my physical health...BOOM! My memories were released and I was hit by reoccurring night terrors and flashbacks of the whole ordeal. This was a particularly tough and harrowing part of my journey.

My flashbacks would hit at any time of the day or night, but the hardest part was waking up in the night thinking I was back in hospital unable to breathe. It would take my brain a while to register where I was and take a breath. I didn't want people to come and see me because I never knew when I'd have a flashback and I was completely out of it when I did. If I had to leave the house I would often have panic attacks. I remember sitting on the floor one time, blocking the front door, shaking uncontrollably because we had to go out. Still not knowing what had put me in hospital in the first place, I also went into a panic about everything, thinking I was going to die from germs or bugs or a common cold. My entire body had just gone into a place of fear, shock and trauma. It was a very delayed reaction to a near loss of life.

My family and friends had been so worried throughout my illness and were pleased to have seen the recent improvements in my physical health, so to see me like this would have really upset them. I kept it to myself for months, avoiding anyone, apart from my (now) husband, as often as possible.

I eventually told my Doctor who diagnosed me with Post-Traumatic Stress Disorder (PTSD) and taught me techniques to help me control my flashbacks. I slowly learnt to manage them and eventually got them under control, but the whole ordeal had shaken me up quite badly.

## The Motivation

At the end of my second year with CFS my Grandad passed away and on his deathbed he said to me "You are better now aren't you dear?". He always wanted so much for me to be better and I couldn't make him sad on his deathbed so I said "yes". It wasn't a lie as I was better than I had been. I could sit up and eat and walk a few metres, even visit him with my family on my good days. So I was very much improved. Just nowhere near recovered.

This little white lie gave me a new push. I had to get better for my Grandad. No matter what it took. I booked myself onto the three-day course offered by the Optimum Health Clinic in London. I had been watching their online videos for over a year and had been desperate to do their course, but felt I wouldn't have been able to cope with the logistics of a three-day stay in London. My new found motivated self didn't care if I slept for two months following the course – I had to go!

The course was just what I needed. It was the helping hand I had been searching for. They were able to help me understand more about what was happening to me medically, some of the underlying reasons why I had CFS and what I could do to recover. This greater understanding eradicated some of the stress and anxiety of living with so many unknowns and enabled me to relax more into my recovery journey. This was a key point in my recovery.

All of the people running the course had previously had CFS and fully recovered. I had never met anyone else who had recovered from CFS (apart from myself the first time) and so meeting these healthy, happy, energetic people really gave me a new lease of hope and confidence in my recovery.

I left the course feeling motivated and enthusiastic. The tools and techniques they taught were fantastic. Over the next few months I was fully committed to putting these tools into practise and saw great improvements in my health as a result.

I then attended the NHS's CFS clinic after being on the waiting list for over a year. I benefitted greatly from the one-to-one counselling where I was able to talk through some of the challenges and stresses of living with CFS.

## The Wellness Warrior

I was now starting to grasp that it was down to me to be my own Wellness Warrior! I had to change my perspective, step up and became my own Champion of Health!

> "ABOVE ALL, BE THE
> HEROINE OF YOUR LIFE,
> NOT THE VICTIM"

> Nora Ephron

I started to see light at the end of the tunnel. I was motivated and feeling optimistic about a recovery. I had new techniques to try, professionals from the clinics advising me and a holistic healer introducing me to a new world. I had a heart full of hope and a mind willing to learn! I started to look forwards towards a brighter future.

I learnt about manifestation and the power of visualisation and positive thinking. I read everything I could get my hands on about the mind-body connection in healing. It opened my eyes to a new perspective on the body!

## The Acceptance

As my eyes opened to a more enlightened world, a calming peace and acceptance came over me. I then did something very important and I forgave my body for being ill. I released the anger associated with having to live with such a debilitating illness. I started to really appreciate my body. I became grateful that my brain had shut down my memories from hospital. I understood that it was trying to protect me as I wouldn't have been able to deal with the mental effects of the trauma whilst physically suffering like I was. I also realised that my body had not 'let me down' by having CFS, it had potentially saved me instead. I gained an understanding that my body is always trying to communicate with me and I recognised that CFS was part of this communication. I started to listen to my body. I befriended it and accepted it for the wonder that it is.

## The Recovery

As the acceptance set in, I started to manage my own health and care for my body in new, more loving, ways. I did meditation and gentle yoga daily. I used crystal therapy to cleanse, boost and protect my energy. I removed electronics such as TV and phones from my life. I got outside in the sunshine every day, even if some days I was only able to make it as far as my door step. I had a healthy diet free from any stresses on the body. I took supplements to help the energy production in my cells. I used the techniques I had learnt to reprogram my mind away from fear and anxiety (brought on by living with CFS), into a setting of health and happiness. Most importantly, I searched for things in life that made me smile, that made my heart sing, that made me laugh. Even a snippet of laughter could erase a whole day of pain. It was the best therapy out there. All of this really helped me to look inwards to what I wanted and to hone into what my body was trying to tell me. There were still a lot of ups and downs, but I saw great improvements and was happy to be heading in the right direction.

I then got married! We had known from the beginning that we wanted to get married, but I had wanted to be strong enough to walk down the aisle unaided before we did. As the improvements to my health continued, we organised a small magical wedding with just a few of our loved ones and it was amazing! A dream come true!

Getting married was a big move for me. I was proud to get through such a big day without crashing and it made me think about all of the other things I could potentially do. My life had been on hold for so long, waiting until I was 'better', but I had now opened the door to a world where I accepted where I was and made the most of the health that I did have. After the wedding I spent a few days recovering then went to the seaside on a little honeymoon. I wasn't able to walk along the seafront or climb the cliffs but I made the most of what I could do and I had a fabulous time.

My health continued to slowly improve and my miracle recovery came a few months later when I went in for some crystal therapy and something shifted in my body. It felt like something energetic was being pulled from my body and when I got down from the table I felt 'strong'. I felt like someone had put my batteries back in and all of my cells had started working again. I felt a strength and stability in my legs I hadn't felt for years. I felt like I could see clearly again. I felt alive. I knew in that instant that this was it - I was free from CFS.

It's difficult to explain how I knew I was finally free from CFS; the buzzing feeling of weakness had just disappeared and been replaced by an inner strength and stability. I felt solid again. Like my body was *whole*. It felt amazing. It's like my body had been gradually healing and this was the final push, the shift in energy needed to take me back to health.

After the crystal therapy, I left my car outside the shop and walked home. It was only a few hundred metres, but it was up hill and I did it with a bounce in my step. I was SO excited. I remember spinning around with my arms in the air and a crazy grin plastered on my face. Passers-by must have thought that I had just won the lottery. I felt like I had. I couldn't wait to get home and tell my husband. I felt alive. I felt free.

As the days went by, my health continued to improve and my excitement and joy at my recovery didn't falter one bit. I continued to bounce around free from pain and exhaustion, and the stability in my body stayed strong. Within a few days I had told my family that I was free from CFS. It was official. This was a big step for me as CFS has so many highs and lows you can often feel that you're on the brink of a recovery just to be smacked back down to earth with a crash. This time however was different, this wasn't a CFS high, this was a true recovery free from CFS. My body had started working again. I was free at last.

Having not moved much for over three years I had lost a lot of muscle mass and was pretty unfit so it took me a while to build up my physical strength, but I took it slowly, with a smile on my face, feeling very blessed indeed.

A few weeks after my recovery I was still feeling great, so we decided to take our dreams off hold and start trying for a baby. I got pregnant straight away, and we haven't looked back since.

## The Now

Being pregnant, followed by the many sleepless nights of parenthood, certainly put my newly recovered body to the test… and I loved it. Every single second of it. I was so grateful for my health and I was so proud of what my body could do. My little boy now keeps me fit; running down the beach, dancing around the kitchen, carrying him for miles when he's fed up of walking in the park. After years of not being able to utilise my body you can imagine how much joy these simple things bring me.

Soon after recovering, I wrote a very long list of all the things I wanted to do with my newfound energy and have absolutely loved ticking them off one by one; Road trips, swimming in the sea, skiing, dancing, tennis, I even dusted off my old netball kit and started playing again. I am so pleased to now feel so healthy, and am very grateful to be living a full and happy life.

Now when I feel tired, it is a normal tiredness that I know will soon pass. I rejoice in how different it feels and am always grateful that it doesn't involve pain and brain fog. I feel "groggy in the normal way" like I wished for in one of my poems.

I now prioritise my health every day and feel blessed that I have learnt so many amazing tools, techniques and lessons to help maintain and improve my health and happiness. I now find purpose in sharing all that I have learnt with others to help them heal. Help them find their own path towards health and become their own Wellness Warrior! I am also in the process of writing another two books to enable me to share all that I have learnt with a wider audience.

My body and I have a new understanding that I listen to any messages it gives me and if, for any reason, I am ignoring these messages, I give my body permission to find a way of making me listen. So now, if I ever have an ache or a pain, I instantly stop and check in with my body. What is it trying to tell me? What can I do to rectify the situation? I am grateful for this new-found relationship I have with my body and I will never neglect it again.

When I look back at my time with CFS, I see the most horrifyingly painful and traumatic time of my life. Yet this image soon gets overshadowed by the thought of the joy, love, peace and acceptance I found along the way. As we part ways I am stronger, happier, healthier and wiser than before and I have gained all of my hearts desires. I now live life from the heart and am surrounded by the most wonderful people who fill my days with love and joy. I am secure and content in who I am and now find love, worth and approval within. I follow my own path in life and enjoy sitting back as I watch it unfold. I wake up grateful every single day for the health I now have, and the life I now live, thanks to all that I have learnt along my journey through the wilderness of CFS.

# THE POEMS

# THE POEMS

The poems are written in chronological order so if read from front to back you will follow the ups and downs of my journey through CFS. Each poem is also given a little context at the back of the book, in the section called 'Setting the Scene'.

Brain fog, weak arms, and the inability to stay awake very long means that reading can often be a challenge for people with CFS. With this in mind, and with the understanding that every day with CFS is different, I have put the poems into categories (see table). Should you choose to dip in and out of the poems, this will help you quickly find a poem that suits your given day. I have also included a list of my favourite poems:

| TOPIC | POEM NUMBER |
|---|---|
| *MY FAVOURITES* | 1, 2, 12, 13, 16, 20, 23, 29, 30, 34, 36, 38, 39, 42, 53, 55, 60, 68, 77, 82, 84, 88, 89, 91, 92, 101, 102, 103, 105 |
| *STRUGGLES* | 1, 2, 4, 8, 12, 13, 14, 15, 16, 17, 18, 21, 22, 23, 29, 30, 34, 35, 36, 37, 72, 73, 79, 80, 82, 85, 86, 89, 91, 92, 93, 98 |
| *PAIN* | 1, 2, 3, 13, 15, 17, 22, 23, 28, 37, 73, 80, 82, 89, 93 |
| *LONELINESS* | 1, 4, 6, 12, 34, 64, 68, 69, 86 |
| *DESPAIR* | 1, 4, 13, 14, 15, 28, 30, 72, 80, 91, 92, 93 |
| *FEAR, ANXIETY & P.T.S.D* | 52, 53, 54, 55, 56, 58, 59, 60, 63, 64, 72, 74, 79, 88 |
| *SADNESS* | 13, 29, 57, 58, 65, 80, 81, 86, 92, 93, 94 |
| *HOPE* | 8, 18, 19, 20, 26, 32, 38, 39, 40, 45, 49, 62, 67, 70, 75, 83, 84, 88, 90, 95, 96, 102, 103 |
| *MOTIVATION* | 15, 25, 26, 31, 39, 84, 88, 89 |
| *PEACE & HAPPINESS* | 5, 19, 20, 26, 42, 43, 44, 46, 47, 48, 49, 50, 66, 67, 75, 76, 100, 101 |
| *FORGIVENESS & ACCEPTANCE* | 60, 61, 66, 67, 68, 78, 84, 86, 98, 101 |
| *HEALING & RECOVERY* | 25, 26, 31, 38, 39, 40, 41, 45, 51, 60, 61, 62, 63, 66, 67, 71, 83, 84, 88, 89, 90, 95, 96, 97, 102, 103, 104, 105 |
| *LOVE & SUPPORT* | 2, 3, 7, 9, 10, 11, 12, 14, 20, 24, 27, 33, 37, 43, 50, 51, 56, 68, 69, 77, 84, 85, 87, 99, 101, 104 |

*1*

# Alone

Today I can't seem to get out of bed
I can't even manage to raise my head
I haven't a clue what's wrong with me
Nobody knows, no one can see

Trapped underneath a ten-tonne truck
I try to move but have no luck
Lightning pain strikes me deep
Nothing I can do but sleep

I crawl to the bathroom on hands and knees
To cater for my basic needs
Need to know what's happening to me
Need to know when I'll be free

Free from this pain, this cloud, this numbness
Free from this prison, this unknown illness
Nobody cares what's going on
They soon stop asking, they soon move on

And I'm left here all alone with me
Barely remembering how to breathe
No longer can I fend for myself
Not with this deteriorating health

Today I can't seem to get out of bed
I can't even manage to raise my head
I haven't a clue what's wrong with me
Nobody knows, no one can see

X

# 2

# Angel Nurse

A few weeks ago I lay in that hospital bed
There were times when they thought that I was dead
In and out of conscious life throughout the week
Unaware of surroundings yet hearing them speak

It was as if my body had given up on me
Let the barriers fall so that pain could run free
Every cell struck by lightning and toxic rain
I lay in a bath of torturous pain

My mind saw a Doctor in the matrix trend
He held out a pill that would make it all end
Take away the pain and release me to death
I reached for the pill and took my last breath

Then the door burst open and a nurse ran in
With a beautiful smile and minstrel skin
"What do you need" she asked from up high
Through the pain I wheezed out 2 words… "to die"

She squeezed my hand through her protective glove
Said "I won't let that happen to you my love
I promise that I'm going to look after you
I'll make sure sweetie that you pull through"

Her words struck my heart then flew to my mind
Reminded me of kindness and love of mankind
On the lonely road to death I had an angel friend
Who turned me around so close to the end

No strength to fight, but enough heart to hope
That this body of mine would fight and could cope
I drifted to sleep blocking the Doctor death curse
Left life in the hands of my Angel Nurse

X

**3**

# *White Light*

White light on the window sill
Here to take me 'cause I'm ill
White light through the window pane
Here to free me from my pain
But no, white light wants me to stay
I'm here to live another day

X

**4**

# *Please Help Me*

I need some help
I can't do this anymore
I'm trying so hard
To fight this stupid war

One step forward
Twenty steps back
I give it all I've got
But don't get any slack

Someone help me
Please make it go away
Rid this ghastly curse
Let me live another day

X

# 5

# Relax for a While

Close your eyes
Release your brow
Feel your face soften
Relax in the now
Unclench your teeth
Feel your face smile
Take a deep breath
And relax for a while
Let your shoulders go
Let them go some more
Sink into your bottom
Sink into the floor
Breathe through your belly
Feel it rise
Let it massage your organs
And restore health inside
Breathe in the goodness
Breathe out the bad
In with the happiness
Out with the sad
Be here in the moment
Be here with yourself
Breathe to happiness
Breathe to health

X

*6*

# *Fingers*

I stare at my fingers
As I lay in bed
They're all I can focus on
So close to my head

Life seems so small
As I exist day by day
I find fascination
In my fingers today

The beautiful skin
Looking so old
A unique pattern
In each crease and fold

Wish I could paint
This scaly dream
Would I do justice
To beauty seen

So big to me now
Never seen before
Beautiful fingers
On my hand I adore

X

# 7

# Poem for My Funeral

Family and friends here today
Thanks for coming to see me away
I'm off on an adventure to pastures new
So I thought I'd write this poem for you

As I write I can't help wonder how I died
Was it something awesome like a free fall skydive
Or was it a boring bus or an African bug
Or did I burst from too much laughter and love?!

As I leave for each adventure, to my folks I always say
"if I don't come home please know, I've loved my life in every way!"
So instead of cry today, please take this chance to celebrate
Drink tequila to my life and eat shed loads of cake!

Please don't be sad today, as you come to see me part
I will be here with you always, right inside your heart
My life may have been short, but it ain't half been fun!
I've lived life to the max and loved everything I've done!

I've had adventures galore, I've had so much fun!
I never imagined that life would be so awesome!
I've dreamt big and been lucky that my dreams have come true
I'm so happy I had the chance to share them with you!

"life is not the amount of breaths" they say
But the moments that take your breath away!"
So despite being cut short, I can officially say
I've lived my life to the full in every way

All that remains of life is loving energy
So know that I've loved you with all that is me
I've had a life full of love, bursting with glee
And that's 'cause you guys have given it to me!

My folks are the best in the whole wide world
So much love and support for their little girl
My big bro, I've looked up to and loved every day
You're the most amazing person in every way!

Gran, grandad, cousins, uncles and aunts
You've made me happy, loved and guided my paths
I love you all dearly and want you all to know
I'll be watching over you like a TV show

My mates, yes you guys and gals out there
Who've mopped my tears and held my spewy hair
You've given me so much laughter and shared so much fun
Promise me you'll live life to the full now I'm gone

When I write this poem I am just me
But my dream man's on his way. Did he make it? Did he?!
It's always been you, the guy of all guys
I'm sending you a lifetime of hugs and smiley eyes

I never feel more happy than when I'm embraced in a hug
Saying I love you as I squeeze you nice and snug
So before I say my last goodbye, I have a favour to ask
Look around at each person today and carry out this task

Whenever your paths cross from this day on
Embrace in a hug, feel loved and strong
Know that I'm hugging you from up above
Sending you smiles and so much love

I'm rambling on as I usually do
So it's time to say goodbye to all of you
God has a heavenly choice waiting for me......
A Porsche full of ketchup or a campervan by the sea!! J

X

*8*

# *Crash Boom Bang*

2 days have been and gone
I'm living on a high
I await the mighty crash
But seem to just get by

I've walked like a zombie
And ached quite a bit
My eyes have stung like hell
But it hasn't really hit

My Doctor's always said
That laughter was the cure
But who knew you could get it
Delivered to your door

I know that soon I'll ache
But in the now I fly
I cuddle up and dream of things
To keep my spirits high

I wish I'd stay this way
But know that I may not
I close my eyes and say my thanks
For every second I've got

X

# 9

## Cry Myself to Sleep

This time 2 months ago, I was crying myself to sleep
Wondering what life was about, as I hung onto it by my teeth
Life had lost all reason, all mission and rhyme
How had I not died? Why did I survive?

Today I cry myself to sleep as I'm overwhelmed with love
I get the message sent to me, from someone up above
This is my time for happiness, to share this love inside
Me and my great big heart no longer need to hide

So as our universe collide, the smiley eyes appear
Beaming like our happy souls, we grin from ear to ear
This is our time, this is our life, our happy ever after
Each day we live, a precious gift, to cherish and look after

We only have one body and one chance to live
Yet a heart has no limit to love that it can give
I've found my special one, of that I have no doubt
So let's enjoy our lives together and make each second count

X

# Daddy

My Daddy is the greatest man in the whole wide world
Every day he makes me feel like the luckiest little girl
He makes problems disappear with one bear hug
He makes me feel safe and makes me feel loved

My kind-hearted Daddy is completely selfless
He looks after me and treats me like a princess
Just one hug from him makes my troubles melt away
I'm happy that I get to hug him every single day

X

# 11

## *Thank You*

You were there for me, when reason was lost
Surviving it all, had come at a cost
I caught your smile in an old memory
Then words brought you to my reality
Your space my sanctuary, you held my life line
Your embrace made you, a saviour of mine
I clung to your light, to shine bright on me
Forever in your debt, I am happy to be

Thank you thank you thank you

X

**12**

# No Name

Sometimes I feel like people don't care
Which is irrational of me and very unfair
I know that they love me and do all that they can
But it's so difficult to really understand

It's a very lonely illness when it has no name
No-one knows someone with it, it's lacking fame
Some are sympathetic but it's hard to empathise
Some don't believe me and I see it in their eyes

I hang onto the solid words that people know
Like 'tropical disease' and 'damaged organs that grow'
I talk of recovery in 'years' so they leave me be
To eradicate the pressure to be bouncy old me

Your palette of friends goes through natural selection
You're left with a good core, a trusty collection
You learn to read people who genuinely care
You learn to release those who can't be there

You're thankful for your family's solid support
You're wiser after any life lessons you are taught
You open up to colour of an enlightened mind
You wish for health and happiness and for life to be kind

You recognise love and let it into your heart
You relinquish control and let others do their part
You're grateful for the people who help you mend
You're grateful for you, you are your new best friend.

X

**13**

# Rip Tide

I'm caught in a rip tide of 30-foot waves
The kind only the wildest surfer braves
Each set brings pain with a forceful pound
Pulling me under and swirling me round

I manage to follow the bubbles with care
Push up to the surface to gasp for air
As I take a breath, it catches my eye
The next tidal wave, 30-foot high

It crashes upon me with the force of a jet
Shattering hopes that I'll shake off the wet
It brings with it new unimaginable pain
It swallows me down, hungry again

The waves continue to take me down
I struggle courageously not to drown
But the tide just drags me out to sea
Further away from my reality

X

# 14

## Too Slow

I'm desperate to get better
But it's happening too slow
Don't leave if it takes too long
I don't want you to go

I'm not getting better quick enough
And I want to come out and play
Before I had no reason
Now I want to live each day!

Sometimes I'm gonna get blue
Sometimes I'm gonna get mad
Sometimes I'm gonna get grumpy
Sometimes I'm gonna be sad

When this happens please don't run
Don't ignore me with a shrug
The only thing that'll make me better
Is a loving special hug

X

**15**

# *So Close*

I am so close to giving up on life
Balancing on the edge of a very sharp knife
The pain is unbearable and I feel so rough
And the very last straw is my poorly tooth

It's pushing me to the edge of the camels back
Like someone's punching me with a mighty whack
It's taken the one thing that keeps me strong
It's taken my smile and it feels so wrong

Hold on in there, I hear me shout
The dentist tomorrow will sort it out
The Doc'll sort your tum on Thursday morn
Soon you'll be back to your poorly norm

Aromatherapy may help your pain
You have nothing to lose and lots to gain
Your milk free tabs may ease it some more
One day you'll be back on that dance floor

Then you just need to build up your strength
Keep it tuned to that healthy wave length
And slowly restore each part of you
You'll be glowing and chilling and bouncy and new

You can do it love, you know you can
You're my brave little lady + I'll hold your hand
Take little steps, just one at a time
You'll get there lovely, you're doing just fine

X

**16**

# Hidden Stars

People who I've met in the last few years
All they see in me is the pain and the tears
They don't know me as the girl I am inside
They only see the struggle I just can't hide
They do not see me as the happy go-getter
The organised, smiley chick, who's got it all together
They see me as the sick girl who's lying in bed
They see me as I struggle to find words in my head
They see me as pathetic, incapable and weak
I offer them a cuppa but can't get up from my seat
I rely on those around me to keep me fed and dry
I rely on those who love me to see that I get by
They don't see my stars, all the things I have done
They only see this shell of a girl that I've become
The sickly shell that hides the girl I am inside
How do I show them that I'm very much alive?!!

X

# 17

# *Laugh-able!*

Laughable! Is that even a word?!
It suit's my week – so totally absurd
The craziness crashes down at full pelt
I'm stuck on a robot conveyor belt

I started with tears as the pain held high
But then I realised I couldn't just cry
The funny side snuck out at last
Then I began to laugh and laugh and laugh

Tablets with milk, to make me ill
Syrup with orange – much worse than the pill
Infected gums, so she cuts out the pain
Only to get infected again

Round 2 with the milk and orange cure
I just don't think I can take any more
My equilibrium lost so quick
Balancing on a banana slip

Shaking nerves and fight or flight
Lost my healing state alright
Aromatherapy chills me a little
But hasn't quite got me out of this pickle!

X

**18**

# Low Poetry

I write these poems
When I'm feeling blue
They help me communicate
My pain with you

But I only seem to write
When I'm feeling crap
I don't want you to think
I always feel like that

These blues are caused by
My limited ability
They're a moment in time
Not what you should label me

I may write of struggles
Of giving up on hope
But I need you to know
I'm strong, and I can cope!!

X

# 19

## Summer Survival

Summer I'd say, begins today
The sun has officially come out to play
Just one wispy cloud, the birds sing out loud
Today is a wonderful day!

The sun won't burn, it's just right to yearn
A gentle breeze whispers by
The flowers bloom, the vitamins boom
We're given a natural high!

I yoga outside, with nothing to hide
On a path to better health
I lie in the sun, listen to music hum
And enjoy being here with myself!

It's days like today, I can honestly say
I'm glad to be alive
I sit here a girl, just part of the world
With a mission to survive

X

# White Butterfly

He just flew by, my white butterfly
On the first sunny day of the year
He rested so close, calming my soul
And the message to me was clear

Everything's going to be OK
I have strength to make it through
To rebuild my body piece by piece
Which I know he'll help me do

He flutters by and catches my eye
And the feeling is hard to explain
(It's like) he pumps me full of faith and hope
To make it through the rain

He's always there when I need him most
Gives me courage to keep spirits high
(It's like) I have a friend to the bitter end
In my beautiful white butterfly

X

# 21

# London Again

On the train, to London again
In search of answers
Through the rain, through the pain
Into the madness

One snores, one's a bore
One eats loudly
I sit in a row, with my hero
My Daddy proudly

I cannot keep, my eyes from sleep
On Dad I rest
I shuffle along, he holds me strong
My Dad's the best

They poke and prod, shake and nod
To find the truth
What could hit, a girl so fit
Just in her youth

They do not know, we have to go
More tests to take
They scan and rub, take lots of blood
I stay awake

Then it's on the train, back home again
I'm far from fine
I do my best, to sleep and rest
Until next time

On the train, to London again
In search of answers
Through the rain, through the pain
Into the madness

X

# 22

## Walking Standing Still

Walking so slow I'm almost standing still
Following the Doctor, does he even know I'm ill?
He sprints down the corridor, expecting me to follow
The speed that I am walking, I may be there tomorrow
I'm clinging to the wall, holding myself straight
Trying not to fall under my skinny see-through weight
He looks over his shoulder and sees that I'm not there
He finds me down the corridor, his face begins to care
She's obviously ill this gal, she's turtling along
Struggling to move herself, she's the opposite of strong
I look into his eyes, I send a silent plea
I'm struggling, I'm hurting, please can you help me!?
I make it to his office and I hang onto his door
I fall back into a chair before I fall to the floor
I take a big breath and I look into his eyes
I pray that he can help me to eradicate my cries.

X

**23**

# Groggy

I'd give anything to wake up one day
Feeling groggy in the normal way
The groggy that washes off under the shower
The groggy that's gone in under an hour

I'm now so tired, I just lie in a heap
My legs ache so much, I just need to sleep
And for a moment I thought I was normal again
That a few hours sleep would erase the pain

That I'd wake up refreshed ready for the day
Jump around and bounce in my normal way
Then reality hits and I remember I'm ill
And no amount of sleep will make me feel well

So instead I go to sleep with the knowledge that I
Will no doubt wake feeling ready to die
A feeling that takes away the energy to shower
The feeling that gets worse with every hour

So all I can do is close my eyes
Get as much rest as possible between the cries
And have faith that I will wake up one day
Feeling groggy again in the normal way

X

# 24

## Crutches

He turned up today, I was still half asleep
I'd had a rough night, so I now slept deep
I woke up with worries and a head full of woe
So he hugged me tight, like he'd never let go

I told him my worries about health and work
How I long to wake without feeling the hurt
I want back in but don't want back here
He gave me his whole undivided ear

He then squeezed me tight as I sobbed and cried
His hug made me instantly better inside
He then pulled away and looked deep in my eyes
It was a look of true love with no disguise

He said he was here now to look after me
His one aim in life was to make me happy
The only thing I need to think about now
Was to get me back to full health somehow

He said he'd be with me each step of the way
He'd help me flush all my worries away
We'd fight it together, give it a right hook
Regardless of the weeks, months, years that it took

Then he put dairy free icing on the cake
Said I had no work related decisions to make
'Cause once I was back to the fit healthy me
I should embrace a year all about me!

A year where I'd find me and do what I love
A year where I'd try things joyful and good
A year where he said he'd look after me
A year that could last 1 year, 2 years or 3!

I felt my troubles just melt away
Could this man be more perfect in any way?
He really does just want to see my smiles
Is God responding to all those nice miles

I'm blessed to have this man by my side
Holding his hand, I have nothing to hide
I can't wait to spend a lifetime together
Grins and smiley eyes forever and ever!

X

# Lean Spleen

Got the train
To London again
Carried around
My ultrasound

Now in pain
With a sleepy brain
Back in bed
To rest my head

Slept shit
Bricking it
In case the rush
I had to push

So in a mard
But tried real hard
To stay awake
For his sake

Doctor ace
Pretty face
Listened good
Did all she could

Explain scan
By previous man
Saw my brain
Spleen in pain

Liver healing
Cirrhosis sealing
Clear to shrink
That I don't drink

Spleen still large
In safety marge
Small compared
To earlier affair

So looking good
Under the hood
What causes panic
Is micro-organic

So all should heal
Long term deal
I fear though
A long way to go

The day will come
When my body has won
Beaten all bugs
With hard work and love

So come on my dear
Have no fear
Stay strong
It won't be long!

X

**26**

# Room to Recover

Last night I went to bed full of worry and woes
This night excitement tingles from head to toes
Last night my health outlook was doom and gloom
This night my organs heal, my body just needs room
Room to heal, room to rest, room to recover well
Room to get over the last few months of living hell
Last night I stress and panic about my future path
This night I feel free to choose things that make me laugh
I'll live a lighter life, less materials and more joy
I'll live a happier life, together with my dream boy
I can rhyme, I can dance, I can help, I can heal
I can be snap happy, capturing things that make me feel
I can rest when I want, I can play with my man
I can do simple things, just because I can
I can look after me and keep me healthy and strong
I can find enough smiles to live happy and long!

X

**27**

# *Lighter*

My whole life lights up when he walks in
Life just feels lighter with the presence of him
He winds up my smile 'til it reaches my eyes
He shrinks down my pain to a manageable size

He makes me feel safe as he hugs me tight
He gives me strength and encouragement to fight
I feel cared for and loved, like it's just meant to be
But most of all I feel it's OK to be me

"The road to recovery may be long" he says
"But we'll make it fun in a million different ways!"
And I know that he means it, I know that it's true
Yes with him by my side, I can make it through

No matter what challenges lay ahead of me now
I know that together we can knock them down
I know that one day I'll get out of this bed
And embrace my new life that lies ahead

So as I lie here all happy, I've a question to ask
How did I survive, without him in my past?
Feels like he's always been here, somewhere within
Every thought of my future takes place next to him

X

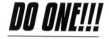

Pain pain go away
Sorry what I mean to say
Is F#@K OFF!! DO ONE!! TAKE A JUMP!!!
I HATE YOUR GUTS!!! YOU F#@KING &%@# !!!

X

**29**

##  Me

I.. miss.. me
Sounds silly but it's true
I miss the me I love to be
I miss being me with you

I miss bouncing up and down
I miss my stupid grin
I miss acting like a little kid
I miss letting laughter in

I'm muffled by my pain
I'm bursting to get free
I'm coma'd by ill health
I'm trapped and I miss me

X

# 30

# Fight from the Floor

I just don't think I can cope anymore
My spirits have officially hit the floor
I'm trying so hard, giving all that I've got
To heal my body, but now I'm full of snot!

I'm fighting a bug and it's knocked me out
I sleep like a sloth and I can't go out
My body aches and my brain is dead
I just can't get my butt out of bed

I normally manage to pick myself up
But the waves keep crashing each way I look
They're battering me and I'm finding it tough
Why does life have to treat me so rough?

I should be happy I fight it myself
No antibiotics just my anti-bug health
The only thought keeping me going
Is that my immune system in finally showing

But it's really hard to keep my smile in place
When the waves keep chucking the bugs in my face
I wake each morning, one thought in my head
I'm tired, make it end, or make me dead.

X

**31**

# Last Train?

On the train
To London again
Chiodini
Lots of pain

Professor smiled
Infections gone
Bugs-nil
Me-one!

Long list
Infections had
No wonder I've
Been going mad

Fought well
Lived to tell
Stories now
And when well

Still to come
The longest road
A motorway
A heavy load

But I'll survive
Fight the fight
Give it hell
Day and night

I will rise
Be well again
Get me through
The tears and pain

One day I
Will run a mile
Yoga queen
Chi Kung smile

Fighting fit
I will be
Walking tall
Back to me!

X

# 32

## Shiny

I have a shiny new book
To celebrate a shiny new me
To match my shiny new liver
And my shiny new spleen

On the path to recovery
Long road ahead
Smiley road of happiness
And lots of time in bed!

This book an empty slate
For the poems that I scribe
Telling stories of recovery
Airing all I feel inside

I have a shiny new book
To celebrate a shiny new me
To match my shiny new liver
And my shiny new spleen

X

## 33

# OXYGEN

I swear I wouldn't breathe if he wasn't in my life
It's like he is my oxygen, I need him to survive
He is the heart that pumps, he is the blood that flows
He is the cells that pass, he is the cell that grows

I swear I wouldn't see if he wasn't there to guide me
I swear I wouldn't hear if he wasn't listening
I swear I wouldn't walk if he didn't hold me upright
I swear I wouldn't sleep if he didn't kiss me goodnight

It's like he is my bible, my morals and my law
He gives my life meaning that it's never had before
It's like he is my body when mine doesn't want to play
He is my other half in every possible way

Without him bones would crumble, I'd lay upon the floor
My heart would stop breathing without him to adore
My brain wouldn't function, not a thought in sight
My soul would escape into the distant light

He's gone for an hour and I find it hard to breathe
Each time that I see him I pray he'll never leave
'Cause I swear I wouldn't breathe if he wasn't in my life
It's like he is my oxygen, I need him to survive

X

**34**

# Dolly

Some days I live in a different universe
It's my coping mechanism to avoid the Hearse
I shut everything out and stare at the wall
It's like I'm a doll and I don't feel at all

I float around when my legs have strength
My mind operates on another wave length
Words don't make it down from my brain
Like a Camel Fubared on a train

I feel so distant from the things I do
I feel so very far away from you
I've stumbled into a parallel universe
I feel bewitched under an ancient curse

I can feel myself do the things I do
I can hear the words when I talk to you
But it's like I'm outside, looking in
Seeing a life I'm no longer living

On the days I look like a spaced out ghost
Don't think you're not loved by the dolly host
She's just slipped away to rebuild and repair
So one day she can ply you with love and care

X

**35**

# *Branded*

Today I bruised my cheek
In my apres dinner sleep
I rested on my knuckle
And now I have to chuckle
'Cause I gave myself a brand
Just by sleeping on my hand
It must have been deep sleep
To leave a bruise upon my cheek

X

# 36

# Simple Decision

Incapable of making a simple decision
Have to think it through with meticulous precision
If I get it wrong my whole life could explode
Every decision is a very heavy load

A simple decision like what to eat
Becomes a life imploding mega feat
Weighing up the consequences of that bite
Will it help you heal or will you suffer tonight?

A simple decision like what to wear
Depends on distance walked or comfort of chair
Is the fabric too heavy, too cold or too tight?
Will it bring on the tears or be just right?

A simple decision like whether to sleep
Bad for your body or a delightful treat?
Surely best to get every hour that you can
If you don't sleep tonight, tomorrow's down the pan

A simple decision like whether to kiss
Can your immune system cope with the germs of his?
Will excitement make you happy and help you heal?
Are you out for the week from the whole ordeal?

A simple decision like whether to walk
Your painful bones feel as brittle as chalk
Should you stretch them out or let them rest?
It's hard to really know what is best

Every decision is a painful fright
Like your whole life rests on choosing right
One wrong decision and your world crashes down
You're back in a slump, crawling around

But each time you fall you come back stronger
Your good days last just a little bit longer
So start to believe in the sound of your voice
Just accept the consequences of a bad choice

You know you better than anyone else
So trust your gut and believe in your health
Give yourself a well-deserved break
Stop thinking so hard and leave a little fate!

X

# 37

## Snap Happy

I'm so sorry that I'm sometimes so snappy
When you ask how I am 'cause you see I'm unhappy
But on nights like tonight when I'm in so much pain
Going home to bed will bring me no gain

The pain will still be there no matter where I am
So I'm trying to ignore it as best as I can
Trying my best to get through a normal day
Smile through the pain and hope it goes away

I love that you care, I love that you ask
But constantly smiling is one hell of a task
So maybe just say once "it's OK to go home"
Then let me go through the rest on my own

When the time comes that I can take no more
You'll be the first I tell 'cause it's you I adore
And I know you'll be fine coming back with me
'Cause I know that you care and you're there for me

Please don't stop caring just 'cause I'm snappy
'Cause it's you my dear that makes me so happy
When I snap I don't mean to get at you
But it's a sign I'm struggling and really need you

X

**38**

# Let the Light In

And she's back in the game!

I feel like I'm ripping through my cocoon
It's been so dark inside, no sun, no moon
I've clawed through the webbing, light's pouring in
It's time to let my butterfly life begin!

I've bounced up and down with a spring in my step
I've enjoyed the rain and got thoroughly wet
When the sun comes out I'll enjoy that too
'Cause this is the season of yellow, not blue

From now on I'm well, just in training you see
To run through the marathon of life that is me!
To enjoy each moment, whatever life chucks
To understand my body is no longer stuck

To bathe in happiness, erase away the pain
Build up my energy and see what I gain
To eat what I want, just 'cause I can
To enjoy my life with my wonderful man!

X

# 39

## My Fairy Godmother day

If I was granted a wish
By my Fairy Godmother
For a perfect day
What would I cover?

I'd wake up early
Full of beans
Bounce out of bed
My smile would beam

I'd turn on the stereo
Play a cheesy tune
And just 'cause I could
I'd dance round the room

I'd open the window
And breathe in the air
Enjoy the view
Without a care

Have a shower
And WASH MY HAIR!
With arms of strength
I'd dry it with flare!

Put on some clothes
Not thinking what'd hurt
My favourite jeans
And my chequered shirt!

I'd run down the stairs
And without any pain
I'd run back up
And do it again!

I'd bounce to the kitchen
Give my Mum a hug
Talk not of illness
But of things we love

I'd go find my Dad
Give him a squeeze
Stand in the garden
In the summer breeze

And without a worry
I'd get in my car
Knowing I was able
To drive real far

I'd pick up my man
Get on the m5
Keep on driving
Til we hit seaside

I'd don my wetsuit
and go for a swim
Grab my board
Attempt surfin

Play for hours
To earn my grub
Of burger and chips
The food of love!

Go for a stroll
Round all the shops
Try loads on
No need to drop

Bounce with excitement
Jump with joy
Holding the hand
Of my handsome boy

Show him I love him
Hug him real tight
No worry of pain
Or skin set alight

Call my folks
Share my day
Call my grands
Send love their way

Write a poem
And get this far
With no sledge hammer
Smashing my arm

Set up a tent
In a site by the sea
Ask my good friends
To come join me

Have BBQ
Make some 'smores'
Cook and relish
In good food galore

Stay up all night
Just 'cause I can
Talking and loving
My beautiful man

Fairy godmother
Please make this true
I believe with my heart
I believe in you

X

# Distraction

First day of the new me
Well a few hours is what I mean
How do I feel pushing through
Bloomin knackered if I tell the truth

But I also feel full of light
And that light just pushed me through the night
I distracted myself when I wanted to fall
I did my best and gave it my all

I'm optimistic that this will work
But I'm realistic as I know it'll hurt
I've organised camping to get me some green
I'll stay at my loves for a change of scene

Who knows what will work or not
But I'm up for the distractions delicious and hot
Brad Pitt following me up the stairs
There for all of my needs and cares

Distraction method is the name I give it
100% is how I'll live it
Living each moment for the immediate grin
Staying awake and not giving in

Day one done and I made it through
Nothing wrong with me, I look normal to you
I keep it strong, I smile through the pain
Do all I can to distract my brain

Been up 13 hours and it's 10 at night
Haven't had a rest but I've had to fight
I've walked up tall and ignored the pain
I look forward to sleep then I'll do it again!

X

# 41

## *Peter Pan*

Day 3
I am still me
To my surprise
I feel alive

Like to ignore
My need to snore
Distracting game
To bury the pain

Right grump
When need to slump
But something to do
Sees me through

Standing straight
Taking the weight
Pains my friend
Til I reach the end

Feel so shoddy
But using my body
'Cause I can
I'm Peter Pan

Make believe
Fly through tress
Believe my grin
The secret to win

Playing games
Cures the lame
Body heat
Cure for sleep

Give it my all
Until I fall
Then get back up
To win this cup

I shall persist
Despite the risk
Wont give in
Have faith in him

Doing swell
Feeling well
Distractions the name
Sleeping's lame!

X

# 42

# Rain When There's Nothing to Do

I love the rain, when you've nothing to do
I love the feel of it falling on you
Drenching your soul and feeding your thirst
Washing away the pain and the dirt

The tension in the air moments before
The sound of the first drop hitting the floor
Cutting the tension, it falls like a knife
Leading the other raindrops to life

The innocent feel as it lands on your face
Not covering up in the speedy rat race
Standing still instead of running home
Standing still getting soaked to the bone

Letting it take you back 20 years
When raindrops wouldn't end in tears
When plans weren't ruined by rain or lightning
In fact they made life more exciting!

So let it land, let it wash your soul
Let it make you again a person who's whole
Let it make you feel alive and well
And relish that awesome post pour smell!

X

# 43

# Angel's Wing

Curled up snug in an angels wing
Not a worry in the world
Feeling safe, supported and loved
Like a cherished little girl

X

**44**

# *Dance*

Today I dance
New tunes on the pod
And I dance....

I dance in the shower
I bop up and down
I dance in the garden
Spinning around

Sun is shining
Heat wave on it's way
Earth's source of energy
Coming my way

I feel so free
In this summer heat
Dancing around
Feeling the beat

I dance
I love to dance
So I dance!

X

## See the light

I feel like I am finally exiting this hell
Like someone has replace my Duracell
There's a long way to go but I can see the light
And my spirits are lifted enough to fight

When I eat food, I feel it do some good
It hits my belly and it does what it should
It gives me energy and stops my shakes
It improves my mood and erases my aches

When I hit a wall, I distract me through
Realising there's more my body can do
I don't need to collapse and fall in a heap
My body is strong and can cope without sleep

Doing things I thought I'd never do again
Meeting people and learning new names
Breaking the boundaries of my enforced solitude
Searching for endorphins to spruce up my mood

Light's flooding in, through tiny cracks
Enough to see but not blind to relapse
I see it now, a future where I'm well
Spirits high that I'll pass through this hell

X

**46**

## Tri

I bounced up and down as he ran into sight
Wolf whistled and screamed with all of my might
Held out a gel to help the next mile
Ran a few steps to capture his smile
Stood in the sun at the finishing line
Didn't pass out, though I sure did in time
Said my hellos to the people that came
Walked like a trooper, not like the lame
I may have passed out when all was done
Slept in the shade now that he had won
But I made it through, a smile on my face
Ran life's triathlon and loved the race!!

X

# 47

## Green

Lying in the park
Surrounded by green
Can't believe I'm here
Living the dream

My lovely Swiss friend
Also lying here
Swiss German tunes
Flow to my ear

Weeping willow
Shades 30 degree heat
Cool green grass
Tickles my feet

Reggae party dance
Round the BBQ
Kids flying kites
Under skies so blue

It's a dream for me
To be here in the sun
Out with my friends
Having chilled out fun

Up and about
My body plays along
Dancing like a fool
To the summer song

So happy inside
That I'm alive to play
On the magical sunshine
Green summer day

So calm inside
With a healing vibe
Feeling so well
Feeling alive!

X

**48**

# Blessed

There's only one word for how I feel
And that's "blessed"
A weekend of pure joy, sunshine
And happiness

I don't care that I cannot move
'Cause my life is now back in its groove
And I am Blessed

I feel like there's so much to share
But I don't know what
The green grass, the heat, the fresh air
The days so hot!

But it's more about the people I'm with
Sharing the weekend we *choose* to live
I am blessed

My bro was so happy it melted my heart
So so nice to see
I was so proud as I saw him pass round
His tongue sticking out at me

I'm blessed I could join in a weekend so great
With my bro, my man and my lovely swiss mate
I am most certainly, totally, excitedly, appreciatedly, wonderfully,
bouncingly, blessed!

X

**49**

# *Corridors*

Corridors
And open doors
Moving parts
And open hearts
Idle chats
And happy hats
Foreign lands
Scorching sands
Flipper fins
And endorphins
Roads ahead
Out of bed
Smiley face
No rat race
Happy me
Being free

X

# Lavender Bush

11 white butterflies on a lavender bush
Fluttering around, no worry, no rush
There to support me through this ride
Through it all, they flutter by my side

X

# Angel Feet

The Lovely Angel at the bottom of my bed
She knows what I'm thinking before it's been said
She sums up my week and the way that I feel
She knows what I'm feeling, she makes it feel real
As I travel through this journey of recovery
She understands what's happening to me
She makes me feel that it's really OK
To feel the things I feel each day
She is my angel and she watches over me
So when I go in it's easy for her to see
Just how I feel and what my body's been through
She sums it up as if she was feeling it too
It makes me feel it's OK to be me
To hear the messages my body gives me
She talks to me and guides me along
She puts all her heart into making me strong
She dishes out wisdom that's perfect for me
To help me through the challenges I see
She talks to the angels and relays what they've said
She's the lovely angel at the bottom of my bed

X

# Another Tunnel

It's like a whole other healing
Has only just begun
Through another tunnel
My body is being spun

Bones and cells are healing
So it opens up my heart
To heal all my emotions
I begin where I start

It's like the cloud has lifted
Up off my daily life
Reborn into the world
Reliving baby's strife

The noises are too loud
The lights are way too bright
I'm surrounded by these people
My body's prepared to fight

It's back up in defence
It's ready to attack
It's pumping the adrenaline
It's having a panic attack

It's struggling to breathe
It's preparing to cry
It's doing what it can
To ensure I don't die

So now I fight my body
And heal with my heart
I'll be guided by my angels
I know they'll do their part

I ask them for guidance
They tell me I'm OK
They hold my ungloved hand
And take me through each day

Through this whole other healing
That's only just begun
I know I'll make it through
This battle will be won!

X

# P.T.S.D

I cry so hard I think I may break
I sob as my heart pounds and my hands shake
I cry as if my world will never mend
Tears and snot just never seem to end
I cry like an abandoned infant might
The reason why still escapes the light
I think it's 'cause it's all a bit much
Reality is slipping from my clutch
I try my best to make it through the day
But I'm out of practice and not in a good way
Something's amiss and life is yet to find
A path which brings a health and peace of mind
I try to live my life as if I care
But all is numb and my street is bare
I need to rebuild my world up high
Find shelter on the streets on which I cry

I cry when I think I'm absolutely fine
But something's pushed me across a line
A noise, a smell, something not quite right
My body feels attacked, my defences up in fright
Survival mode kicks in and tries to save me
Releases adrenaline, pumps it round my body
It becomes too much and I begin to cry
'Cause to my mind this means I'm going to die

My whole world balances on the edge of a knife
Whilst I walk the tightrope of my precious life
A feather flutters like a hurricane
Pushing me off balance over the edge again
Something so simple, the end of the world for me
The Doctor gave it a name of P.T.S.D
I associate this with war, that sounds about right
'Cause I've spent so long frightened in this fight
I will now face my fear and do what I need to do
To win this battle and bring my body through

X

**54**

# *Cry*

Let it all out and
Have a good cry
You'll soon be asking
Yourself why

Why was I crying
Why was I sad
I'm feeling much better
It can't be that bad

X

# Waking Up

Waking up was the hardest part
The PTSD
Being out of it was easier
Like it wasn't happening to me

It's all coming back to me
A bit at a time
The state of my mental health
Turns on a dime

Everything is so so loud
My mind just cannot cope
The sound of sports on TV
Makes me cry so hard I choke

The thought of leaving the house
Has me shaking like a leaf
Lost in my disabilities
I have no self-belief

Too many people talking
Is as loud as a bomb
Exploding my fragile brain
That's been asleep too long

I sit in the corner
Closing off my senses
Try get back inside myself
I've lost all my defences

Arms wrapped around my knees
I rock myself assured
I cry because it's all too much
I'm literally floored

I start to remember
My hospital bed
How I gave up on the breath
I was very nearly dead

I remember stopping breathing
The sound of that loud beep
I remember how I wanted
To drift into endless sleep

I wish my brain asleep
In it's survival trance again
Where everything is quiet and numb
And my only thought was pain

X

# Day 5

It's now day five
I'm glad to be alive
Had hospital flashbacks
When breathing was lax

Had a good cry
When you called tonight
Needed it so much
Your voice I could touch

You make me feel whole
You fill up my soul
Can't wait til you're home
It's no fun here alone

X

# 57

# Weeping Willow

Weeping willow
Why so sad?

X

# Basic Breath

It was too much hard work to muster a breath
My body was sloping slowly to death
It'd given up on life and was ready to leave
Then Dad shook my arm, making me breathe

I heard the Doctor ask a nurse
Why the sats monitor was screaming a curse
She said not to worry it sometimes went wrong
I thought 'oh crap I'm not gonna last long'

I think my body was ready to quit
I'd take one breath and not need the next hit
I'd wait it out 'til I heard a sound
Which prompted my brain to take the next round

The beeps bought back the Doctor guy
He looked at me with his own eye
Saw I was in a deathly dream
Put me on an oxygen machine

It forced the air inside of me
So I didn't need to do it consciously
I look back and thank god for this
It saved my life with an angel kiss

That night they took blood from a painful wrist
Tested for oxygen, said I was at risk
I couldn't survive with so little oxygen
So I was woken from sleep by two Doctor men

They said I needed to remember to breathe
Consciously think of it and never give in
In and out, in and out
It hurt so much but I'd not live without

So I opened my throat and ignored the pain
Consciously breathed again and again
Remembered as each one came to a close
To take the next big breath, in through my nose

When I think of it now it doesn't seem real
To forget how to breathe is a really big deal
To not be able to do the single one thing
We absolutely must do to keep on living

It comes naturally to us and we don't need to think
To breathe is as unconsciously done as to blink
So think of the state my body must've been in
To have forgotten to breathe out and in!

So now I take each breath with pride
Thank my angels for being by my side
Thank the night Doctors for visiting me
Thank my breath for making me me

X

# Forgiveness

I've made a new friend
In this body of mine
We've a new understanding
That things are just fine

We're living each day
Together as we are
If we hold hands together
We'll make it far

I understand now that
It's looking after me
Doing what's best for
My mind and body

It shut my mind down
'Cause I'd never had coped
With this emotional healing
When physically broke

But now that I'm stronger
It's opening again
To deal with all of
My emotional pain

So I work through each week
A day at a time
Dealing with these
Emotions of mine

Flashback and nightmares
of Doctor death
choosing to die
taking my last breath

giving up
listening to the beep
fading away
lying in a heap

but I work through these issues
my body and me
and I understand why
I set my mind free

Free to rest
Whilst my body repaired
Rest well to wake up
Ready to care

And now each week
I feel a little more together
Every day gets easier
Every day bets better

My angel helps me
A blessing each week
Aligning my chakras
And pummelling my feet

Anyway the meaning
Of this poem is to be
That I forgive myself
My body and me

Forgive it for the things
We've been through this year
The things it had to say
I needed to hear

Forgive it for shutting
Down my mind
I see this now as
an act that was kind

And as I now wake
To a life so raw
I'm getting me back
A me that is pure

I see a future ahead
Of wholeness and calm
Body and mind together
Riding any storm

X

# Just the Way I Am

I forgive you body
For all that I have blamed you for
I'm OK that you're not bouncing around like you used to
I need to use this time to get in touch with my mind
To listen to myself and my body
To live each moment of the peaceful, calm and whole life I lead
My body and I are wonderful just as we are right now
We're not meant to be anywhere else, doing anything else, in any other state
We are perfect just the way we are
Just the way I am
Right here
Right now
I am me
And I love me
Just as I am

X

# Wherever

Lights are shining
Path is widening
Getting there
Wherever there is

X

# Heard

Today I feel heard
Don't feel so absurd
My fears have been aired
My traumas shared

I voiced the flashback
My Doctor fell smack
Of my fears and my tears
I've held onto for years

A visualisation he gave
To make me no longer a slave
To thoughts of my death
Giving up on the breath

I now move it to a screen
Make it fuzzy like a dream
Dull colours to black and white
Turn volume down to just slight

This makes it less emotional
And kicks in my brains rational
It detaches it from me
So I can then let it go free

X

**64**

# *In Case I Don't Wake*

Will I awake
When morning comes?
Heart is pounding
Left arm is numb

Think that it's just
My adrenaline
But can't be sure
If hearts giving in

If I die in the night
Please know that I
Love you to bits
My family and guy

X

# *Empty Inside*

Today I feel low
And why I don't know
I feel empty inside
And I just cannot hide
From this feeling of blue
Of darkness so true
I think it's not me
Yet it is what I see
But why I don't know
Why I'm feeling so low
I just do

I can't reason, can't hide
This deep feeling inside
I thought it had passed
But I've not seen the last
Of this side to the story
The shadow so gory
But I know from the past
That this feeling won't last
I shall just ride this wave
Onto sunnier days
....and I will
....I have to

X

# *Releasing the Fears*

Releasing the fears
Of this time of year

Letting it go
Letting it flow

Feelings of peace
Of calm, of quiet
Take over the tension
The noise, the riot

Releasing the fear
I'll never be well
Releasing my ties
To this untimely hell

Freeing my soul
To take the next step
Stop looking back
Let's try to forget

X

# 67

## The Revealing of Me

I lie on my angel's bed
She knows what's inside my head

A sadness comes over me
Then I release and set it free

I'm now lying in a field of grass
Breeze blowing as daisies dance

I lie on my back looking up at a tree
I begin to see the hidden real me

Light as air I feel my feet
Tension released from calfy meat

I look forward to what this may bring
A revealing of me in time for spring

My journey has only just begun
My lovely song is yet to be sung

I'm light, I'm airy, I'm happy, I'm calm
I look to a future with me in my arms

X

# Not Alone

All together
A unit
On a journey
Together
Together
Not alone
But together
I really needed to get that sorted in my head
Together
Not alone
I am not alone
I did not go through it alone
We all went through it together
It "happened" to me
But it also happened to us all
I get it now
I am not alone
I am not alone
I
Am
Not
Alone

X

# My Hug

On the anniversary of the day I nearly passed
I got some release from this loneliness at last
The days that followed were lonely and blue
Not a soul in the world I could really talk to
Then you went quiet and felt so far away
I thought you didn't care but you corrected that today

"It was the most destroying thing to see
You were lying there dying in front of me
The bouncy girl that normally does in my head
Is lying like a corpse in this hospital bed
It ate me up inside and I couldn't let it go
Didn't know what to say, didn't know how to show
It cut me up deep so I'd come sit with you
I didn't sleep for months, didn't know what to do
I saw you disappear into that living hell
And it took over a year for you to look well
There's no words to describe how this made me feel
I just wanted you well and to finally heal
I know I went quiet but it's all I could do
But you know deep inside that I really love you
Life's not worth living with you not here
I'm so glad you didn't die this time last year"

I needed to hear that. I needed that hug
That lasted so long, as snug as a bug
I needed you always here by my side
And a year to this day I now realise
You were here all along but hurting so bad
And you just couldn't tell me 'cause I was so sad
So you wait til I'm strong to tell me your story
And it completes my heart, the truth so gory.
You were there by my side, living it with me
Today I feel better, I'm loved, not lonely

X

# 70

## Feb Celebrations

The celebrations are over
I've had so much fun
I love to celebrate life
I may just carry on

Carry on celebrating
Each and every day
Make every day special
In each and every way

Just have that joyful attitude
That each day's a gift
That you've done well to survive 'til now
Without getting heavens lift

So make the most of each day
Walk through life in a haze
Of happiness and celebrations
Make the most of your days

Everyday a 'survival day'
A party for 'beating the bugs'
Full of family and friends
Full of love and hugs

X

**71**

# Tubes

Tubes coming out my nose
What a problem does it pose?
Well I just can't swallow food
Which doesn't really help my mood
When you've been told to shove your face
So you chew and chew without grace
You attempt to then swallow it down
But it rips out your nose, you say ow!
You realise there's something in your throat
Survival mode makes you choke
You try to cough it all right up
But it's stuck real tight like a glove
You realise it's lodged in your throat
Try to breathe but realise it won't
There's something stuffed up your nose
Making your throat feel like it's closed
So you try to fight with the wire
See what it is and release it like fire
Try to wrap around your head
You can breathe, take a breath, you're not dead
"I can breathe; this is weird" I then say
What a rather extraordinary day!
I have to look in the mirror to believe
What it is, that is stuck inside me

This happened and only two seconds passed
How long your life threatening can last
It's just a wire going up my nose
But my what problems it does pose

X

**72**

# Please Just End

Oh my god
Will this day please just end!
It's been one crap sandwich
A nice filling of a friend

I woke up shattered
My brain was full of fog
The hospital had wiped me out
All I could smell was dog!

I ripped my new trousers
Whilst looking for some tea
I shouted at my boyfriend
For just saying hello to me!

I went to the Docs
Wanted to say good things
But it wasn't true today
I was really suffering

My whole body felt
Completely seething mad
Raging from the inside out
It was oozing from me bad!

I think if I'm honest
It's linked to my PTSD
'Cause the nurse said something
That had an effect on me

I walked in to her room
And she started to talk to me
That's all I remember
Then my brain shut down on me

It all felt numb again
All fogged up inside
Just like it used to do
When it was trying to hide

I think it may be now
Trying to shake me awake
But I wish that it would hurry up
'Cause it's really really late

And I just want to sleep
make this day end at last
I can't cope any more
I need this in my past

So please let me close my eyes
And drift off into sleep
Say goodbye to today
Let tomorrow be a treat!

X

**73**

# A Treat Indeed

Tomorrow was a treat indeed
I woke up in insufferable pain
Read my book and yoga'd my yoga
Tried to make it through the rain

The difference today was in me
I laughed instead of cried
I saw the fun in my hideous pain
The blues decided to hide

I went to see a 3D movie
Left my glasses in my draw
I proper threw a toddler fit
It was like my final straw

But at least today I laughed
I let the anger fade to none
And now it's time to go to sleep
Another day has gone

I wonder what tomorrow will bring

X

**74**

# *So Loud*

It's the noise that's gets to me
Since I came out of my cloud
There's some things I can't cope with
They're just so friggin loud!

I don't mean the parties or discos
The horns of cars or trains
There's just these certain noises
That will send me to my grave

The commentators of sports
Raising blood pressure so high
Too many people talking at once
Fighting for their piece of pie

The washing machine going
When my brain is trying to think
The sound of dishes clashing
In the kitchen sink

And when my flashbacks hit
They don't ever disappear
Until I turn the volume down
And can no longer hear

As I swizzle the volume nob
On my old fashioned TV
I feel my heartbeat slow
And I breath nice and slowly

I feel me melt back to earth
When I eradicate the sound
Back to a land of calm and peace
Two feet firmly on the ground

So please don't talk at once
And don't watch sports on TV
Don't talk when the radios on
And don't multitask with me

And when I lose my mind
And I flashback to my past
Let me picture it on TV
And turn the volume down real fast

I promise I'll soon be better
Although today I am still whole
I'm happy with my progress
And happiness is my goal

X

# 75

# Floaty Flowery

I want to live in a world that's light and bright and flowery and misty
A world where you can run in a field in a floaty white dress and just laugh
A world that's a little clouded, even sheltered, and naive and innocent,
and full of sunshine and unicorns and care bears and sunshine people.
I think a little make believe is OK.
Whatever gets us through the day.
I want to see the good in things
I want to forgive the bad
I want to relax, be free, be gentle, be kind and be at peace.
In my happy floaty colourful peaceful world!

X

**76**

# By the Sea

Sitting by the sea
My favourite place to be
Waves gently fold
Breeze blowing bold
Wrapped up warm in bear
Without a single care
I'm sitting by the sea
It's my favourite place to be

X

# 77

# Perfectly Normal

You organised the trip
Around my limited abilities
You didn't even mention it
As if you had no difficulties

You'd really thought about it
It worked seamlessly well
You made me feel as if I wasn't
Dragging others through my hell

We drove from spot to spot
So I didn't have to walk
We stopped for some sight seeing
Upon the cliffs of chalk

We caught all of the action
A hindrance I didn't feel
I felt perfectly normal
And that's a really big deal

So thanks for your effort Mum
It will never be forgotten
If you can't walk when old
I'll be sure to spoil you rotten

X

**78**

# Life Has Begun

There are lots of things I can't explain
Like the disappearing Malaysian plane
Like the Bermuda Triangle, the Mary Celeste
Things like this put my mind to the test

I watched a Blacklist it spooked me out
So I started talking to Dad all about
Life on earth and life on the stars
Are we all alone? Is there life on Mars?

He talked of atoms and carbon based
Bodies of ours that we just seem to waste
It made me feel like we're so so small
And like life doesn't really matter at all

But for whatever reason we're here right now
Loved ones are gathered all around
And it matters to them what happens to me
And as they're my world, it matters to me

This is not meant to be a sad note from me
I'm just questioning what life really should be
My perspective has changed so much this last year
What was gold before I no longer hold dear

So I need to rearrange my vision to be
Because I want a life where I'm just…happy
Surrounded by loved ones to share my glee
At being alive, at being healthy

At being free to do our hearts desire
At having time to stoke the fire
To keep life burning through the night
So life can go on just as it might

So what I'm really trying to say
Is I now search for happiness every single day
I no longer wait for the next thing to come
I'm living for today, my life has begun!

X

**79**

# Cloudy Day Unbeknownst to Me

It's weird how my head was stuck in a cloud
Noises were muffled
Thoughts were slow
Things moved slower
But I didn't know
Not til the cloud lifted and I was back in fresh air
Did I realise how I'd just not been there!
I'd been absent. Lost. Muffled and muted
My brain had been replaced with cotton wool
My body was in survival mode
and I obviously didn't need those senses to survive life
in the protection of my sick bed!
But I didn't know I was in a cloud
'Cause I didn't have the ability to know
I just knew when I came back to the land of the living and the cloud lifted
But others knew I was stuck in a cloud
They can tell me the exact date I started to come out of it
I remember it too
It was a dark day
And only darker days followed
It was like being born
Leaving the safe muffled protection of your mother's womb
To come out into the loud bright scary world

Where things moved and attacked all your senses
Yes! That's it. I was reborn
This is my second life
Me 2.0

X

# 80

## *Tough*

My angels are putting me firmly in my place
I'm ahead of myself, making my journey a race
I was starting to feel like I could see the end in sight
So I started to plan and get excited as one might
Then I hit a brick wall and it crashes down on me
I'm struggling so much and it's really hurting me
My body aches and burns like it's been beaten by the hulk
I forgot my meds one day and it's gone into a sulk
I've thrown it all off kilter and I feel utterly shite
I'm so totally tired and I'm trying with all my might
To smile my way through this and get out the other side
But with it comes depression and memories I try to hide
I like to live each day as if it's life anew
And not try to think of all the crap that I've been through
But feeling all this pain just brings reality back to me
I may be getting better but there's still a long road for me
So don't plan too much and live for each day
Try to smile and get through this very painful day
Tomorrow might be better, like it already has been
And you know what you are aiming for, you know what you have seen
Just take this placid journey, one step at a time
And remember that this journey is 100% mine.
You can make it as you like, happy, sad or blue
How wonderful your day will be, is only down to you

X

# 81

## Be Gone Old Blue

So dark and so blue
These feelings are true
Here with me now
Don't know why or how

But I want fully rid
Of this emotional unbliss
Dunno what it is
But I can't handle it!

A wave of despair
Not a single tiny care
No way to express
This deep down sadness

I hold in the tears
And with it my fears
Can't reason why
This feeling's inside

It's so dark and so blue
Not black, just blue
Logic hibernates
It's a sad sorry state

I know I'm in pain
That it's hurting again
And it's getting to me
I just want to be free

Free from this illness
Free from this stillness
I want to move on
It's gone on so long

That light up ahead
Now fades in my head
As the pain floods back in
And I feel weak within

Legs giving way
On a nice sunny day
I just want to dance
Thought now was my chance

Until waves crash on me
This relentless sea
Draggin' me far
I long for the calm

For the placid sea
Gently swaying me
Through an ordinary day
In an ordinary way

Be gone the darkness
Bring back the happiness
Yellow, not blue
Be gone, Old Blue!

X

# Bus. Stop.

You wake up in the morning
You've been hit by a bus
You try not to cry
Not to whinge, make a fuss

But every bone is broken
Every muscle smashed
Every nerve on fire
How long will this last?

You wake up the next morning
The darkness has dispersed
You still ache and hurt
But there's less need to curse!

X

# 83

## In Touch with Me

I smell stuff I have never smelt
I feel stuff I have never felt
I see stuff I have never seen
I think stuff I could only dream

X

# Warrior

I am my own way forward
The challenged and the challenger
I am the champion of my health
I am my wellness warrior!!

X

**85**

## *Alike*

I'm sorry that I upset you
We are just so alike
We want everyone to be happy
Everything to be just right

I just don't like to think
That I'm letting anyone down
'Cause my legs don't work so well
I can no longer get around

And I know you never mind
And you try to make me feel
Like I'm OK just the way I am
So sorry I made a big deal

You are so so special to me
I'm so lucky to have you here
To care for me and love me lots
And fill my life with cheer

You always care so much
You have such a great big heart
You always make me feel OK
You've supported me from the start

I don't know what I'd do
Without you standing by my side
So thanks for being so bloomin' great
And coming along for the ride.

X

**86**

# Cheap

I Feel kinda blue
Like I sort of been used
Like I've talked myself down
To people around

I feel sort of cheap
People see what they see
Without knowing the past
They see through me like glass

They don't know what it's like
To always have to fight
To make it through each day
In a patient calm way

Considering my plight
I think I'm doing alright
I think I'm doing well
In fact I'm doing swell

I think it's just me
I care what people see
I'm starting to release
And gain an inner peace

I give myself a hard time
Which is a fault of mine
Don't want them to believe
That this illness is me

I have chronic fatigue
From a tropical disease
I have nothing to prove
I have nothing to lose

So just let people think
Whatever they think
All that matters to me
Is inside I'm happy

I have hopes and dreams
Despite what it seems
I'll live in the now
I'll make it somehow

To the other side
Where I don't hurt inside
Strong as can be
I'll feel more like me

Where dreams can come true
'Cause my illness is through
But for now it's just me
Being all I can be!

X

**87**

# Unconditional

You look after me like it's no trouble at all
You are there to pick me up when I fall
You are always there unconditionally
You make me feel it's OK to be me.

Thank you

X

# *The Fears of a Fretter*

Today's the day my outlook has changed
I see going forward in a million different ways
The future looks bright bought on by the orange
Leaving fears behind my future has changed
I don't feel ill, I feel ready to get better
I shan't be held back by fears of a fretter
I shall look forward to my life ahead
To happiness, to kids, to getting wed
I'm excited inside, the fear leaves my back
Possibilities bring joy, no longer a life trap
Today's the day my outlook has changed
Today's the first of a million different days!

X

**89**

# Better and Worse

When the good days get better
The bad days get worse
You have heightened awareness
Of this illness curse
You remember the joy
That the good days hold
Making bad day's pain
Stand out in bold
You love the life of
Your upwards trend
Making it harder
When the graph does bend
But hold on in there
You can make it through
To a shining bright light
To a shimmering new you

X

# I See That I Can See

I really can't believe this
But I think that I can see
I didn't know that I was blind
But someone's just cured me!!
We've finally cleared the fog
That's been weighing down on me
Or maybe I'm just looking up
Not looking down at me!
I hope this feeling lasts forever
I want to always see
The beauty of the universe
The beauty that is me

X

**91**

# Giving In

Today I've officially had enough
Whether I live or die I don't give a f#@k!
I can't be arsed to live like this
It's doing my head in, it's taking the piss
I could scream all day at the slightest thing
The door bell ringing or the dog whimpering
I'm so cheesed off so stay out of my way
Today's written off in everyway
I've listened to reasoning I already know
I've understood things they're trying to show
But I just want to know what to freakin' do
To make me walk around all day like you
This half-life I'm living is wearing thin
And today I just feel like giving in!

X

# 92

# Struggling

I'm struggling at the moment
Feel lost
Stuck
I have no reason to wake up in the morning
My life mission is to 'make it through the day'
That's pathetic
My good days are getting better
Making my bad days worse
I just watched TV for first time in 2 months!
I needed a distraction from my overwhelming sadness and despair
I watched overboard
Goldie never fails to make me smile
So maybe if I could just distract myself a bit more…?
Continual distractions to keep my mind off being blue
But surely that's just 'making it through the day'?
I'm trying to be positive
Not flooding my body with negative messages
It's kinda working
Until it doesn't
Like today
I had a lovely day yesterday and was on a high
It never crossed my mind that today wouldn't be wonderful too
So to wake up unable to move is a shock
An unwelcomed shock
A huge disappointment

Making me feel more depressed
I need a reason for living
All the books say take the first step in what you want
I want a baby
There is no first step in that
So I'm lost
I'm trying to motivate myself to do something I can.
Maybe pottery
But my hearts not in it
What do I really want to do with myself?
Even a short term goal would be better than nothing
But I have nothing
I'm empty
I'm lost
I just want to make it through the day
And that's depressing
I need a light to shine on me
In me
Around me
Wherever
Just a light
I need a reason to smile
Logically I could list hundreds of reasons to smile right now
I am very lucky
But right now I'm blue
Right now I can't stop crying
So what good is a list
I could use the paper to mop up my tears
I just need to find my zest for life again
My joie de vivre
My raison d'etre
The thing that makes me excited to wake up in the morning
And I need to shed this gloomy cloud
I think I'm clearing so that's good
But be done with it already

I've held a positive head throughout my debacle
This healing journey of mine
But I feel nowhere near the end of this journey
In fact I feel like this is the beginning
So I get why I need to take it slow
But right now I need to smile
No matter how slow it goes
I need to smile
Just smile

X

**93**

# Rock Bottom

I shall never forget
The bottom of the pit
Empty darkness and pain
All alone where I sit

Empty of feelings
Struggling to live
I realised I had
Nothing left to give

No joy left inside
No hope to cling to
No smile left in sight
Just empty dark blue

The good thing of bottom
Only 2 ways out
Off Beachy Head
Or back up the spout

Luckily my angels
Gave reason to hope
So I start to go up
Climbing this rope

But I need never forget
This rock bottom feeling
As I carry on with joy
In my journey of healing

X

**94**

# Goodbye

We all stood in a row
Waving him goodbye
Just like Grandad's done for us
A million different times

We clung onto each other
In a solid knitted wall
A unit of family love
So none of us would fall

I got to say my goodbyes
To his empty vessel of life
But I know that he could hear me
And he heard my prayers last night

I'll miss you so much grandad
You were the best a man could be
You've shown me love and care and pride
You've shaped me into me

So you go rest in peace now
Up with God so true
You'll always be deep in our hearts
We'll look after Gran for you

X

**95**

# *Back to London Again*

On the train
To London again
This time for something more fun

Next to my man
Playing cards 'cause we can
We'll keep playing 'til I've won

On the Train
To London again
The CFS Clinic I'll be in

Teaching me tips
To give CFS the kick
This battle I soon will win!

X

# 96

## Just What I Needed

The CFS clinic
Was just what I needed
They understood me
And the struggles I deal with

They threw me a life line
I felt heard, I felt hope
They taught me new things
That will now help me cope

My questions are answered
My fears are forgotten
I've seen the survivors
Not festered or rotten

I've seen with my eyes
Them bouncing with glee
I know one day soon
That spring will find me

An important discovery
Was the reasoning behind
Getting ill in the first place
I've answered my why

Now on to the future
New tricks I shall play
This body of mine
Will be healthy some day!

X

**97**

# *Stop Right Now*

Stop right now, ask yourself why
You're travelling this path again

'Cause it's the most trodden path?
Shame it's a path to pain

Turn off your GPS short cuts
Get out your map of paper

Take the long windy scenic route
You'll be thanking yourself later

X

# 98

# Benefits of Having a Cold

So I have a cold and it's clear to see
That there is something wrong with me
People understand and sympathise
They can see my red nose and puffy eyes
They give me a break and don't pester me
They leave me alone and let me be
They know I'll get better so they needn't ask
They know I'll soon be back up to the task

I know too that it soon will pass
I give myself a break and relax at last
Know how to treat a cold, common is it's name
So I don't need to play an impossible game
Of trying to work out what's wrong with me
Of proving to others I try to be healthy
I just chill out and let my immune system get 'em
I don't feel guilty for not 'trying' to get better

Why can't I feel like this every day
I suffer yet I beat myself up each day
For not being able to cure myself
For not being able to return to good health
Maybe I need to learn from this bug
And relax every day, give myself a hug
Care for me, love me, give myself a break
Believe that I'll one day wake up feeling great

X

**99**

# 10 Things I Love About You

I love the way you love me
The way you make me feel

I love the way you look at me
And make everything feel real

I love the way your hearts so big
It can be felt from outer space

I love the way on our first hug
I felt your big heart race

I love the way your gorgeous grin
Reaches up to your smiley eyes

I love the way your kindness
Reaches everyone under the skies

I love the way you know me
Almost better than myself

I love the way you care for me
In sickness and in health

I love the way you tell me
You've won life's lottery

But most of all I love the way
You've chosen to spend your life
with me!

X

# Laughter

Today I laughed so hard I couldn't stop
I was on the phone to Chop and Wok
I couldn't stop laughing as I ordered the food
What a feeling! What an awesome mood!
I laughed so hard that I actually cried
Couldn't stop no matter how hard I tried
Every word ended in a girly giggle
Worked my stomach muscle in the middle
Can't remember when I last laughed like this
Not a worry in the world! It's utter bliss!!

X

**101**

# I'm OK with Me

"I'm OK with me" mirror
I see truth in my eyes
I say the words "I love you"
I choke and start to cry

Why is it so hard to say?
I love me. I really do.
But the girl staring at you now
Has she ever said that to you?

You've never stopped long enough
To look at her and say
You're perfect just the way you are
Perfect in every way

So when you judge her harshly
Or let others judge her too
Take her to the mirror and say
"You're OK and I love you!"

X

## Could This Be It?

Could this be it
Could this be real
Can I now walk
Can I now feel

Strength in my legs
Strength in my bones
And just 'cause I can
I walk my way home

Could this be me
Strong once again
Free from this curse
Free from this pain

I pray that I'm right
Strength to be me
To live a full life
Healthy and free!

X

# 103

# Me and My Body

I have a body!!!!
Attached to my head!!!!
An actual body!!!!
That's out of bed!!!!

I can't believe it
Not felt for so long
This feeling of oneness
I'm feeling so strong

I'm going to love
My body so much
Savour each feeling
Feel every touch

I'll love every inch of it
It's really mine
I'll look after you
We're gonna be fine

I'll love you body
The way only I can
I'll keep you healthy
I'll hold your hand

Woohoooooooooooo

I have a body!!!!
Attached to my head!!!!
An actual body!!!!
That's out of bed!!!!

X

# 104

## Crystals and Angels

Thank you crystals
For all that you did
You pulled out the curse
From the places it hid

Thank you my angel
For healing me so
Where I'd be without you
I just do not know

I'm now free from illness
I've regained my strength
My brain now works
On a healthy wave length

I'll forever be grateful
And cherish you true
Thanks crystals and angel
For all that you do

X

# Looking Back

Looking back, I only see
The good things that have happened to me
The joy I've felt these last 3 years
Overpowers the tears and fears
The truth of it came out of the blue
All that I ever dreamed has come true!!
A man who I love with all of my heart
A home to live in so we're never apart
The chance to live a life of leisure
The reduction of all the endless pressure
A family that now knows the true me
The same happy soul without the need
And the greatest dream to come from above
Is to have a baby with a man that I love
I see that happening now I feel so strong
I'm so excited, I've waited so long
And all this has happened in a rocky time
You'd presume would be a bad memory of mine
But I'm grateful for all that this journey has given
All my dreams have come true. I can now start livin!

Woohoooooooooo!!

Thank you. Thank you. Thank you.

X

# SETTING THE SCENE

# SETTING THE SCENE

1. **Alone**
   This was the first poem that I wrote on this journey with CFS. Written just a few weeks into my illness. I was lying in bed literally unable to move. I couldn't even get to the bathroom. I was feeling immense pressure to get better instantly so I could go back to work. I had recently moved to a new area to be closer to work, so felt very isolated and alone, away from my family and friends with no one to come and help 'cater to my basic needs'. It was a very scary time.

2. **Angel Nurse**
   I didn't write another poem after the first one until I came out of hospital a few months later. I had nearly passed away a couple of times in hospital and I just couldn't get my head round it all. I kept replaying my white light moments (my close calls) and also the scenario that I write about in this poem. My Doctor visited me at home when I came out of hospital and I knew he would understand but I couldn't find the words to explain to him how I felt and what I went through. This poem was written whilst I was trying to get my head round it all.

   Shortly after writing this, my mind shut down these memories and although I knew something drastic had happened I couldn't remember all of the details. I later realised this was my body's way of protecting me as I wasn't strong enough to process it at this time.

I can only presume that the third verse of this poem was an hallucination as I doubt a doctor came along and offered me an out! I really remember the nurse though – I always wanted to send her a copy of this poem so that she could understand what an important part she played in me pulling through – I didn't have the energy to find her at the time – so if you're reading this – this is for you – thank you.

3.  **White Light**
    Trying to make sense of my white light moments in hospital.

4.  **Please Help Me**
    This is me pleading for someone to help me. I was trying SO hard to get better and I just wanted to know if I was even heading in the right direction. I was desperate for someone to come and tell me what to do.

5.  **Relax for a While**
    I was meditating lots at this point. I really enjoyed doing a body scan as it gave my mind something to concentrate on which reduced my mind chatter. I came up with this poem whilst doing a body scan one day.

6.  **Fingers**
    I remember lying in bed day after day, unable to move, my mind numb. Days went by where I just stared at my fingers. I began to see a beauty in each skin cell. It was quite fascinating having a different perspective of the body. I was desperate to photograph the skin cells but my camera was too heavy for me to pick up so it came out in poetry instead. My arms were often so weak and in so much pain that writing was agony, resulting in poems that were often illegible to anyone but myself.

7. **Poem for My Funeral**
I couldn't shake the feeling of how life had nearly been taken from me. I knew I was lucky to come out of hospital alive and as my health seemed to be deteriorating instead of improving I worried that if something like that happened again I may not live to tell the tale. I started to worry about all of the people I would leave behind and how they would feel. My family were still processing nearly losing me and were all still in shock. I needed them to know that if I died I'd had a good life, in fact a great life, so they needn't be sad. I wrote this poem and put it in my parent's filing cabinet next to my will.

8. **Crash Boom Bang**
During my journey I met my (now) husband. Or re-met him as I'd known him for years. As soon as he heard how poorly I was, he came round to see me and never left. He sat by my bed every night after work, just holding my hand. He made me smile and he made me laugh – he bought sunshine and hope into my life. This was written 2 days after I'd stayed up late one night talking to him. The excitement and adrenaline made me feel more 'with it' than normal which was awesome. I crashed literally minutes after writing this poem.

9. **Cry Myself to Sleep**
I was bursting with love when I wrote this. I couldn't believe that my (now) hubby was in my life. My dream man was by my side. I had this huge feeling that the universe was trying to tell me that this was my time now! My time to thrive. My time to survive. I was literally BURSTING at the seams with love.

10. **Daddy**
My folks were amazing when I moved home. My Dad had just retired so he looked after me most days. He was an absolute legend. Not once did he complain or question anything and I felt so blessed to have him there with me. I felt so loved, like a little girl again – I remember feeling so much love for him that I had to get it out on paper.

11.   **Thank You**
When I came out of hospital, I felt like I couldn't really talk honestly to anyone about how close I had come to dying and how much it had scared me. My family were all in a bit of shock after my near loss and I really didn't want to upset them further. One day an old friend's cheerful face came to mind and even though I hadn't seen him for years I just felt guided to talk to him. He was a magical friend to me and I was able to let loose some of the thoughts running around my mind.

At the time of writing this poem I didn't even remember what had happened in hospital but I remembered that he had been there for me. I don't think he ever understood the gravitas of his friendship and how much of a life-line he was for me. I wrote this poem for him, looking back, to say thank you.

12.   **No Name**
This had been a tough month. It felt like people were bored of me being ill now and just needed me to get better. I was struggling to explain to people what was going on. They were OK for the first few months after I was in hospital but then no one really understood why I wasn't getting better. One of my best mates was very absent and it hurt so much that she wasn't there for me when I needed her most.

13.   **Rip Tide**
This is one of my favourite poems. It pulls so many heart strings. I remember sitting on the sofa unable to stop crying. I literally couldn't stop. Mum tried to help and talk to me, but I couldn't speak. There were no words. Only tears. And they kept coming. Not gentle tears. Full on snotty sobs. It was all just too much! I felt like I couldn't cope anymore. Mum asked what I needed and I just used my hands to mime the action for pen and paper. Rhythmic words were repeating over and over in my head and I had to get them out. This for me is one of the most emotional

poems of my journey. I had lost all hope and couldn't see a way out.

14. **Too Slow**
I could see a great life ahead of me with my (now) hubby. I was desperate to get there and start enjoying life.

15. **So Close**
This was written on a particularly bad day. When you're struggling to make it through each day something as small as a bad tooth can literally push you over the edge. I felt like the whole world was closing in on me. Burying me. This was a bit of a vent with a hint of much needed self-motivation. A great example of how the process of poetry could take me from despair to hope in just a few lines.

16. **Hidden Stars**
I was meeting a lot of my (now) hubby's friends for the first time in the first year that I was poorly. Being bedbound, ghostly white and unable to get up on my own wasn't the kind of first impression I wanted to give and it really upset me that they only knew me as a sick girl. I used to use every ounce of my energy to look as normal and be as smiley as possible when people came round. I'd then be completely wiped out for days.

17. **Laugh-able!**
This was written at the point when you can cry no more and you have to see the funny side of life.

18. **Low Poetry**
I felt like I was constantly writing about the bad times, so I wrote this for my (now) husband to let him know I was strong and shouldn't be defined by these low moments.

19. **Summer Survival**
This was a good day. I felt happy to be alive.

20. **White Butterfly**

In moments of struggle there is often a white butterfly that flutters by. I see him as my sign that everything is ok.

21. **London Again**

I had to go down to London to the Hospital for Tropical Disease every week or two whilst they tried to find out what was wrong with me. I usually had so many emotions flowing through me I'd end up writing a poem on the train there or back. These trips were absolutely gruelling. They completely wiped me out.

22. **Walking Standing Still**

This was again from one of my trips to the hospital. I remember dragging myself around the corridors holding onto the bit that sticks out of the wall that hides all the electrical wires. It was recommended that I have a wheel chair but I feared that once I got into one I'd never get out again.

23. **Groggy**

Waking up feeling horrific again, I dreamt of waking up like a normal person: Groggy, tired, but able to shake yourself out of it in minutes.

24. **Crutches**

This was a big day for me. It was the day I realised I wasn't alone and that I had someone by my side every step of the way. I was finally living on a two-way street of unconditional love. It felt epic!

I also released a lot of pressure this day. I had previously been working towards a recovery that involved going straight back into work in a life which my soul had obviously been trying to escape. Deciding that the day I fully recovered was going to be the first day in a year of joy, excitement and exploration, now that was something to look forward to! The weight that lifted off my shoulders that day was immense!

25. **Lean Spleen**

This was another trip to the hospital in London. Tests showed that my liver was healing and my spleen was out of the danger zone, which was fantastic! I was still no closer to working out what had caused the damage, but a healing liver was definitely worth celebrating.

26. **Room to Recover**

This was me dreaming of the future now that physical signs of the tropical disease were healing. I had been living with the fear that the tropical disease would take another shot at killing me and succeed the next time. So I think this was written on the first day I actually started to believe I could survive and be fully better one day.

27. **Lighter**

This was written about my (now) husband. He really was my rock and he brought joy into my life. I actually wrote hundreds of poems about love throughout these 3 years, but I only put a select few into this book that were relevant to this journey. The rest of them have gone into a separate book about my poetic journey to Mr Right.

28. **DO ONE!!!**

A very bad day. I was in so much pain and it made me angry! Really angry! Excuse the language. The last word was unprintable so you'll have to use your imagination.

29. **Me**

It was hard not being my normal self. It wasn't my old life I missed. I just missed feeling like me. I wanted to feel alive again.

30. **Fight from the Floor**

A self-explanatory tough day.

31. **Last Train?**

This is the last time I went to the Hospital for Tropical Disease. Whatever tropical disease had attacked my liver would remain a mystery now that it was healing. I was pleased that they had signed me off because it meant I was out of the danger zone. I was also secretly gutted, because my hope for them finding something they could cure quickly was lost. I had a long road ahead of me.

32. **Shiny**

I was on the train back from London and had just bought a new note book. This was a poem to start the new book because I find it hard to write the first words on a perfectly clean book. It's like the first scuff on your new trainers.

33. **OXYGEN**

This was about my (now) husband. I felt like he was carrying me both metaphorically and physically and I felt very blessed for his love and support.

34. **Dolly**

I often felt so numb I didn't really know what was going on. The problem with this is you don't really know you're numb until you come out of your cloud for just a moment and you realise you haven't really been present. This was written in one of those moments. I never intentionally wrote any poems for my (now) husband but often the thoughts/worries in my head would be aimed at him so the poems were just written that way. I would often read them to him which he found really useful as it helped him understand what was going on with me.

35. **Branded**

A random little poem. I often had to sleep after a meal because it was so exhausting just being up and eating. I woke up from this nap with a bruise on my cheek as I'd fallen asleep really fast, just leaning on my hand. I actually wasn't going to include this poem but it surprised me how many people who suffer from CFS related to it and enjoyed seeing the humour in the situation.

36. **Simple Decision**

When you have CFS, Every…Single…Thing… has an effect on how you feel. Not just in that second but within the next few days. If I needed to wash my hair, I had to do it two days before the time I needed it done so I could recover in time. Choosing what to wear was a nightmare because everything hurt when it touched my skin. When writing this I was fed up of the anxiety involved in making decisions that should be so simple. I will never take the simple things like this for granted again.

37. **Snap Happy**

I was trying my best this night to be normal. I think we'd gone to the cinema. My (now) hubby had carried me in. I remember being in excruciating pain but I was trying my best to ignore it. My thought was that I would be in pain no matter where I was so I may as well enjoy watching the film whilst I was here. My (now) hubby was concerned because he could see how much pain I was in, but I just wanted to be normal for one night, so I snapped at him – this was me processing the thoughts in my head later.

38. **Let the Light In**

A good day. I can't remember why but I love reading it. There were many times throughout my journey when I was having a good day, that I would try to convince myself that I was better and I just needed to build up my strength. This was one of those times.

39. **My Fairy Godmother Day**

On the day I wrote this poem, my Doctor asked me a question: "If your Fairy Godmother came to visit you and said she could grant you your perfect day, what would it be?". I had to be specific and very detailed. At the time I didn't really understand why I was doing it, but then it all became clear! It sparked some kind of passion and joy within me. Gave me things to look forward to. Just by writing my dream day I was able to think about things differently and implement little bits of it into my daily life. For example, I'd said I wanted to wake up, and dance around my bedroom to some cheesy music (sounds simple but something I would never have had the energy to do), so the next morning I remember waking up and whilst struggling to move I asked my Mum to put some cheesy music on the stereo and I lay in bed with a smile on my face. I may not have been dancing, but I was half way there, and I was dancing in my head. I slowly put bits of the dream day into my life and it gave me a new joy for living. I absolutely loved this! It was a fantastic tactic – thanks Doc.

40. **Distraction**
The next thing my Doctor recommended was to distract myself. So when I felt like I was going to crash, I should distract myself with something that made me happy, something that got my endorphins flowing. This was the poem from the first day that I tried it.

41. **Peter Pan**
This is about the distraction method as mentioned in the above poem. It worked really well for a few days but then I think I took it too far and so I just kept crashing. I took what I could from it and learnt to look for the joy in things, but also learnt to recognise when my body really needed to rest.

42. **Rain When There's Nothing to Do**
I was in the garden when it started to rain and as I never got anywhere fast I got caught in a proper downfall and I LOVED it! Reminded me of when I was a kid. So free.

43. **Angels Wing**
I had a lot of trouble sleeping at this stage and so I used to say this to myself over and over to lull myself to sleep. It was a lovely feeling of comfort and safety.

44.  **Dance**

Looking back at this I laugh. I remember this day clearly and in my mind I had DANCED! Like really danced. In reality, I had just stood in the sunny garden, with my arms in the air, moving my hips a little bit. This is not what most people would call dancing, but at the time it was a huge step for me, and it felt amazing! I was so proud!

45.  **See the light**

A glimmer of hope. I think I had new meds which had helped my stomach and I actually felt like I had eaten, I felt full for the first time in a year! I'd begun to smile again thanks to the Fairy Godmother exercise. I'd started to seek out joyful things. I may not have been able to do much physically but I was learning to enjoy what I could do and this made a big difference to my mental state.

46.  **Tri**

As a result of my "Fairy Godmother" wish, I went CAMPING! My Brother and (now) hubby organised it all so I literally just had to sit there and enjoy it! We went away just for one night to watch my Brother do a triathlon. My (now) hubby carried me to the start line and we stayed there cheering my bro on each time he came past on his laps. It was so much fun for me to be out in the fresh air doing something. I felt alive! The second it was over I just crashed. I literally sank to the floor where I lay, in a field full of hotdog vans and track fencing. I woke up a few hours later – it was dark and my mate was just sitting there next to me on the grass. All of the burger vans had gone and the course had been packed up. The field was completely empty; it was like waking up in a different world. I was so proud of what I had accomplished that day. It was the first day I felt like I was really living. My physical health was still the same, but I was happier and that is the difference between dark and light. Thanks Doc for showing me that I just had to view my situation differently to be happy.

47. **Green**
This was written lying in the campsite field on the same weekend as above. There were people all around us having parties and kids running around. I even had a little sway to some music. It was just what I needed.

48. **Blessed**
This was also from the same weekend as above. My new-found gratefulness for what I had was overwhelming.

49. **Corridors**
This is probably the only poem that I read back and don't remember where I wrote it or why.

50. **Lavender Bush**
Again my butterflies were there for me. (see 20)

51. **Angel Feet**
This was about the Aromatherapist I found to help ease the pain in my legs. She became one of the most important people in my recovery. I went on to have Reflexology, Angelic Reiki and Crystal Therapy. The treatments really helped me shift my energy into a better space.

52. **Another Tunnel**
This is the first poem from what I would call my "dark times". It was like my body had physically begun to heal a little, so my mind could come out of the cloud in which it had been hiding. Everything just became too much. Even someone talking to me was too loud, my senses were in overdrive. It hit me very hard.

53. **P.T.S.D**
Once I explained the symptoms to the Doctor he said I had P.T.S.D which made sense after everything I had gone through. It was like I had just been born and the world was too much for my senses. At the time I didn't tell anyone apart from my (now)

husband and my Doctor as I didn't want anyone to worry. I would have worried if I'd have seen me like this. My family and friends had been through enough already.

54. **Cry**
Again trying to process the tears and fears

55. **Waking Up**
This is when my flashbacks to my close calls in hospital started. I had completely blocked the whole ordeal from my mind. I knew I had been in hospital but had blocked out the specifics until now. The flashbacks just kept on coming and I was re-living it again and again and again. Day and night.

There was a break in my poetry here for a few months. Not even my poems were helping me process this. It was a dark time.

56. **Day 5**
My (now) hubby had gone away for a few weeks to attend a family wedding abroad. I wasn't well enough to travel and was missing him lots. This was a tough day as he was normally there when I woke up in the night with flashbacks.

57. **Weeping Willow**
There was a weeping willow in the garden that I could see from my bed. It felt like a friend through these tough times.

58. **Wounded**
Self-explanatory. After another tough night

59. **Basic Breath**
Another poem about my flashbacks to my time in hospital. Remembering lying there in peace not needing to breathe as everything just went calm. I think I realised how poorly I must have been to have needed to consciously force myself to breathe. The memory hit me hard.

60. **Forgiveness**
The last few months had been a massive learning process for me. At this point I had started to really appreciate my body. I felt that it had protected me by blanking out my memories after hospital and making my mind numb. I would not have been able to process everything mentally whilst unable to move physically. It would have been too much. My new found appreciation for my body was immense. I forgave my body for all we had been through and tried to move on together. Whole.

61. **Just the Way I Am**
A rarity for me to not rhyme. Processing my thoughts.

62. **Wherever**
A moment of hope

63. **Heard**
My Doc came to save the day here. My flashbacks had gotten out of control so I went to see my Doctor and told him about them. He gave me some techniques to help distance myself from the images in my flashbacks. Over time these slowly began to work and I was able to get a grasp on reality again. Thanks Doc.

64. **In Case I Don't Wake**
Since being in hospital, I was scared at how quickly life could be taken from you. I felt really poorly the night I wrote this and I was on my own. It pulled on my fear that I'd not have time to tell people how much I loved them before I died.

65. **Empty Inside**
A wave of sadness.

66. **Releasing the Fears**
It was getting close to the time of year I had been in hospital last year. I felt it was time to release the hold it had over me. The fear it had me living in.

67. **The Revealing of Me**
At one of my crystal therapy sessions I had a big breakthrough and released some sadness and fear that had been holding me still. It was a great feeling!

68. **Not Alone**
It's hard to think of those around you when you're using all of your energy trying to survive. I was now starting to realise that it wasn't just me who was going through this journey. My loved ones were going through it with me. I wasn't alone.

69. **My Hug**
The anniversary of me being in hospital was a massive deal to me – I honestly didn't think I'd survive the year and so I was overwhelmingly chuffed that I had. I asked a couple of close friends to come round to help me celebrate. People that had really been there for me over the year. I just wanted to say a big thank you to them.

During this party my friend explained what it was like for him when I was poorly and it made me realise that he had been through a healing journey too after a big shock seeing me like that.

70. **Feb Celebrations**
About the party mentioned above.

71. **Tubes**
This poem always makes me and my (now) hubby chuckle as it was so amusing at the time. It is a little poem written comically about some wires I had up my nose going into my stomach to check out what was going on in there as I still wasn't digesting food as I should. It was the weirdest sensation ever.

72. **Please Just End**
A self-explanatory bad day

73. **A Treat Indeed**
Written the following day, I think I hit a limit on pain and just had to laugh. I was able to get out of bed and go to the cinema though so not such a bad day looking back.

74. **So Loud**
Noise was a massive trigger for my PTSD.

75. **Floaty Flowery**
A dream of mine!

76. **By the Sea**
My family took me on a much needed trip to the seaside!

77. **Perfectly Normal**
Whilst at the seaside my brother was doing an organised run across the cliffs and I presumed I would just have to sit in one spot and see him once as he passed, but my Mum surprised me with some legendary organisation. Knowing I couldn't walk more than a few metres she worked out where we could drive to so we could see him several times. This meant so much to me because it was organised as if my abilities were the norm so I didn't feel left behind. I was so grateful and I really appreciated it and had a lovely day.

78. **Life Has Begun**
Just a bit of pondering on the meaning of life and how my perceptions had changed since being ill.

79. **Cloudy Day Unbeknownst to Me**
This is looking back at how I came out of the 'cloud' and I hadn't even realised I'd been in one to begin with. I was trying to get my head around it all.

80. **Tough**
Another dip in my rollercoaster ride

81. **Be Gone Old Blue**

This was my first wave of real depression. I had never felt so dark. So hopeless. So lost. Since being ill I had often felt sad and frustrated and like I wanted to give up, but I had never experienced real depression until this point. I remember when I started to come out of it that I had such huge empathy for anyone suffering from depression. I only had it for a few days on this occasion but wow, it was horrible. I had always been such an optimist about everything in life and had never experienced anything even in the same realm as this.

82. **Bus. Stop.**

I wrote this in two parts. The first two verses one day and then the third verse the next morning.

83. **In Touch with Me**

Awakening a little more. Regaining all my senses

84. **Warrior**

A motivational verse. I had realised that I was the only one who could get me better. I couldn't rely on anyone to fix me. I was my own Wellness Warrior!

85. **Alike**

I was meant to be going to a family event but I couldn't get out of bed. A family member didn't understand why I couldn't move today yet had been able to get out of bed the day before. They didn't make a fuss but whatever they said hit a nerve with me because I was already annoyed at my body for letting me down. This was me apologising.

What we know about how energy works with healthy people doesn't fit with CFS. You just crash at random times and don't really know why, and one day you can do something that you're physically incapable of doing the next. It's so hard for people with CFS to get their head around, let alone those around them.

86. **Cheap**

I remember writing this after talking to some medical students who wanted to know more about CFS. They were perfectly nice, but like so many others, they looked at me in that way that said 'surely you can just get out of bed and get on with life?!'. It's a look of disbelief. And it hurts. It deeply hurts. It hurts every bit of you when you're trying sooooooo hard to get better and you wish with all your heart you didn't feel like this but you do. You then find yourself in the position of trying to *prove* to them that you're ill. You give examples of how bad you are. When really the last thing you want to be talking about is how bad you feel. It's such a shame because I truly believe that this pressure of having to prove to people that you're ill, only adds to your illness, because of the stress and hurt that it causes. And let's face it, people with CFS are hurting enough.

87. **Unconditional**

I was very grateful for the unconditional love of my parents. It must have been hard for them to see me so poorly, and having just opened my eyes to how much they had been suffering, I was overwhelmingly grateful for how they had looked after me.

88. **The Fears of a Fretter**

I was very motivated this day to try to move on from my "dark times". I had my flashbacks under control and was a little less anxious and sensitive to noise.

89. **Better and Worse**

Self-explanatory.

90. **I See That I Can See**

This sounds very metaphorical but it wasn't, I could genuinely see things clearer. Like a fog had lifted.

91.    **Giving In**
       I did a lot of emotional clearing at this time. I think I was clearing
       the anger of being poorly. The poem is pretty self-explanatory.
       Please excuse the language!

92.    **Struggling**
       A note to myself. I needed something to cling onto to help me go
       forward. I felt very stuck. I felt like I couldn't really do anything
       because I didn't have the energy or the physical capabilities, but
       my brain was working again and I was desperate to move forward
       with my life.

93.    **Rock Bottom**
       Here I'm looking back at the bottom, being grateful for moving
       on up. I suppose I was still trying to get my head around it all.

94.    **Goodbye**
       This was a very sad time for me as my Grandad passed away and
       he was my hero. On his death bed his last question to me was "you
       are better now aren't you dear?". I didn't want to upset him so I
       told a white lie and said "yes". Following his death, I was more
       determined than ever to get better, no matter what it took. For
       him. To make him happy and to make my last words to him not
       a lie.

95.    **Back to London Again**
       This poem is about the train journey to London to go to the
       Optimal Health Clinic. It was the first time I had made the
       journey to London since my visits to the Hospital for Tropical
       Disease. I had been reluctant to go to the clinic prior to this point
       as I felt I wouldn't have been able to cope with the logistics of a
       three-day course. The travel, sleeping, eating and getting about.
       My new found motivated self didn't let this stop me! My awesome
       hubby-to-be came with me to help, we planned it all out with
       taxi's and hotels and food and everything I could possibly need.

96. **Just What I Needed**

This poem is about my excitement after my visit to the Optimum Health Clinic. I felt motivated and enthusiastic about all of the techniques I had learnt. Most of all I felt heard. I felt like I wasn't alone. I felt like I had found some experts who could help me on my journey.

The course was fab. It taught me what was happening to me medically, what I could do to recover and some of the underlying reasons why I had CFS. Once you know this it is so much easier to move on with your recovery, as you stop giving yourself a hard time and the pressure to understand is released. I'd recommend it to anyone suffering from CFS. It's not an instant cure but it's an open door to a land of understanding where you have techniques and methods to help cure yourself.

97. **Stop Right Now**

This was written about one of the techniques I had learnt at the Optimum Health Clinic to help rewire the brain to a healthy wavelength. It was really helping me.

98. **Benefits of Having a Cold**

I had a stinking cold over Christmas this year and it actually made me relax. When people asked how I was I said "I have a cold" and they instantly understood, sympathised and then left me alone to recover. This was not just the reaction of others, but it was mine too. I relaxed and took care of myself and gave my body the time it needed to heal from the cold. I decided it was time to give myself a break and transfer this relaxed attitude across to my life with CFS.

99. **10 Things I Love About You**

I wrote this poem to read to my husband at our wedding. We had wanted to get married since we first got together but had put it on hold until I was 'better'. I wanted to be able to stay awake for the whole day and walk down the aisle without my legs giving way.

Since my Grandad's death I had been trying to search for the joy in everything, trying to get 'un-stuck'. I didn't want the illness to define me anymore. I wanted to take my life off hold. I wanted to start living. I now felt like I was strong enough to enjoy the day, so we organised a lovely little wedding with just a couple of friends and family. It was a dream come true. It was magical. It felt like a new beginning. It opened up a world of potential; If I was strong enough to get married, what else could I do!?!

100. **Laughter**

A strange thing to write about but I hadn't laughed like that in years. It was a magical moment for me.

101. **I'm OK with Me**

This is about a technique I learnt from my therapist at the NHS CFS clinic. She taught me to look in the mirror and tell myself that everything was OK, that I was OK with myself and that I loved myself. At first I couldn't understand why she wanted me to do this because I thought I already believed all of these things anyway, but the first time I did it I actually couldn't get the words out and started to cry. To look yourself in the eye and tell yourself these things is actually quite amazing. We so often look externally for our approval and love and self-worth, but to find this internally brings such a wonderful, relaxing feeling of peace.

102. **Could This Be It?**

A few months later I had a Crystal Therapy session and something shifted! It felt like something energetic was being pulled from my body. It was particularly painful but when I got up from the table I felt like I had strength in my legs for the first time in three years! It was amazing! I even left my car at the place and walked home (granted it was only a few hundred metres up the road but this was more than I had walked in years!). This poem was me when I got home praying that this recovery was for real.

103. **Me and My Body**

This was written soon after the above. I was so happy to feel solid again!

104. **Crystals and Angels**

I felt so grateful to my Angel lady for doing the crystal session that helped me regain my strength. I had been slowly improving in recent months and this was the final thing that really rid my body of CFS and helped me feel whole again.

105. **Looking Back**

This is such an important poem. I really believe that there is a reason people get ill and for me I believe I got CFS to slow me down enough to really start living a full life. I used to think the more you did the better you were living, but the opposite is true. I was living so fast, and doing so much, I was missing everything. I was forced to slow down and from it I gained all of my hearts desires! Thank you CFS xxx

# GOODBYE FROM YOUR BOOK

# GOODBYE FROM YOUR BOOK

*Dear Friend,*

*Thank you for following this poetic journey through CFS.*

*For those of you with CFS, I hope that these poems have made you feel heard and understood. Remember that you are not alone; there are others out there going through the same as you and there are also people out there who can help. There is hope. I'm gutted that CFS found you. Were you lost too? What is CFS trying to tell you? Look inside your heart to find your answers. Become your own Wellness Warrior, your own Champion of Health. Find your own unique path to a healthier happier you. Let laughter eradicate the pain, let joy eradicate the despair and let love eradicate the loneliness.*

*I hope that this book has given you a few short cuts on your journey to a healthier and happier life. If you'd like some more guidance, keep an eye out for my author's new books coming soon. The first is a short eBook called 'To my BFF with CFS' detailing the honest unfiltered advice she'd give to her friends if they had CFS. It is the book that she wishes someone had written for her during her illness. The second book is called 'Cracks of Light', which will show you simple steps to bring light, joy, health and happiness into your life. This book will be written for everyone, but will have been founded upon her journey through CFS, so will have particular significance to you. Be sure* to sign up to her mailing list to find out the release dates! (details at the back of the book)

For those of you who have loved ones with CFS, thank you. Supporting someone with CFS can sometimes be difficult, as every day is different in this world of unknowns. Finding the words to describe the pain, fatigue and loneliness of CFS is often too difficult a task for someone with little energy and major brain fog. I therefore hope that these poems have helped shed some light on their potential journey. Remember that sometimes just showing up with a smiling face, a sympathetic ear and compassionate eyes is all that is needed. This alone can bring light into the darkest of days. If you can also help them find their peace, their acceptance and their joy, whilst giving them the space and support to discover, and relax into, their own unique path to recovery, you will be making the world of difference to their journey. Thank you for reading me and thank you for all that you do.

For those of you treating people with CFS, my hope is that these poems have highlighted some of their potential daily struggles. I hope that this assists you in helping them find their unique holistic path to recovery. I thank you for taking the time to read me and I thank you for all that you do in helping those with CFS.

For those of you who are new to CFS, I hope that these poems have given you an insight into the debilitating lonely world of CFS. I hope that they have given CFS a voice, where it often sits alone in silence. Thank you for investing the time in reading me. My hope is that if you ever come across someone with CFS you will be accepting of their situation and do what you can to support them through their journey. The more people who can do this, the lesser the grasp CFS will have over us, and the quicker people will recover, so spread the word!

It has been good to share this journey with you.
Remember I am here for you on your everydays.
I am your book.

      Love always
          Your Book x

# ACKNOWLEDGEMENTS

# ACKNOWLEDGEMENTS

There are so many people I would like to thank here because without the love and the support of those around me I don't know where I'd be. I am so thankful to all the people in my life who helped me through my journey with CFS. Whether you cared for me when I was unable to care for myself or just showed up with a friendly face when I needed it most, I will forever be grateful. Thank you. There are also some very special people, who I have met post-CFS, who were integral to the making of this book. Whether you brought me editing genius, rallying support or laughter and joy, I thank you.

A big shout out goes to the following people:

Thanks to my darling husband Dom. You made every day worth living. No matter how dark the days, you would always be there to bring in the light with your massive heart and smiley eyes. Thank you for your endless supply of compassion, patience and love for me when I needed it most. Thank you for your unwavering support through it all and thank you for the encouragement and freedom to write this book. You are, and always will be, my hero.

Thanks to my awesome son. My little legend. You made my ultimate dream come true. Thank you for your patience whilst Mummy types away, for your fun-loving perspective on everything, for your ingenious ways of putting my newly recovered body to the test, and for your never ending ability to make me smile! You make me so proud every day. You are the light of my life and I love you loads xxx

Thanks to my amazing parents who have loved and supported me my entire life and held my hand through this journey. Thank you for welcoming me home with open arms when all was lost. Thank you for taking care of me when I couldn't. Thank you for having an open mind and accepting me for all that I am. A huge thanks goes to Mum for your constant love, for always going that extra mile when organising anything for me and for letting me know it was ok to not be ok. A big shout out goes to Dad for keeping me breathing in the ER and for your unwavering patience and love whilst looking after me each day. A massive thanks to both of you for helping me entertain the little legend whilst I finished this book!

Thanks to my Angel Nic. There are not enough words in the world to describe how grateful I am to have you in my life. You have shown me the light, guided me down a path towards spiritual joy and introduced me to such a magical world that fills me with wonder and delight every day. You have taught me so much and for that, I will forever be grateful. You are a magical healer, a wonderful teacher, a caring mentor and a loving friend. Thank you, thank you, thank you.

Thanks to Doctor Miller for the loving care and support you have given me throughout both my times with CFS and beyond. Thank you for always believing me, believing in me and for always knowing what to say. Thank you for your gentle nudges towards an enlightened life, for helping me find my joy, for saving me from my flashbacks, and for always filling your waiting room with poetic beauty. You will find your footprints throughout these poems as you helped carve out my path toward a healthier happier me :)

Thanks to my amazing big bro for your pure awesomeness and constant love. Thanks for always being there and for organising amazing things like our camping trip. Thanks for always making me smile when I needed it most and thanks for your hugs: - their rarity makes them all the more special :)

Thanks to my soul sister K'Nikki for your unconditional love and never-ending support. Thanks for always being on hand to provide such amazing help, encouragement and editing genius. I am so happy to have found you. Muchos Love :)

Thanks to my beautiful Sarah Rose for doing such an amazing job on the cover of this book. You captured the true essence of the book in just one image and for that I am truly grateful. Thanks also for holding my hand whenever our paths intertwined.

Thanks to Ally for your lifelong love, hugs and friendship. Thanks for dropping everything and coming to see me when I needed you most.

Thanks to Marco for making your second home here with me and for travelling so far just to sit by my side.

Thanks to Carla for bringing the cinema to me, Sarah for the non-walking walks in the park, Kib for the time-defying friendship, Gibbo for the saving embrace, Aimee for the hospital companionship, Steph for the comradery and KTD for the loving care packages.

Thanks to the Rozzier's for your friendship and Murphy walks, the Prices for your love and happy visits, the Woodall's for your loving care and rainbow cakes, and the Walker-Grahams for your loving friendship.

Thanks to Joni, Nats, H, Jenni, Claire, Shell, Skip, G-Man and the Hills for your visits and love that kept me smiling and entertained throughout my journey.

Thanks to my Grandad who started this journey with me but didn't quite see me cross the finishing line. You spurred me on towards getting the help I needed. Thank you. You were the best a man could be.

Thanks to my Gran who crossed the finishing line with me but couldn't stay to see this book. Thank you for helping me write my first ever poem. I feel your amazing strength with me every day.

Thanks to the in-laws for making me feel it was ok to be ill and for your great advice along the way. Above all, thanks for raising my adorable husband to be the kind, loving person that he is - without him this would have been a much bleaker story.

Thanks to Murph for your constant love and companionship. Thanks for being slow on your feet just to make me feel better :) Miss you loads. Sorry you didn't make it to see this book but thanks for seeing me through to the end of the chapter.

Thanks to Alex Howard for starting the Optimum Health Clinic (OHC) and for sharing all of his CFS knowledge and wisdom with the world – a great deal of the knowledge and vocab I have on CFS comes from my time at the clinic so you will find it sprinkled throughout this book. Thanks also to Nikkie and Jess at the OHC for holding my hand through the course and beyond.

Thanks to Linda for your friendship and Chi Kung wisdom, to Liz for your scrumptious nutritional wisdom and to Kim at the NHS CFS clinic for your mind wisdom and much needed conversations.

Thanks to Richard for your welcoming smile and endless supply of beautiful healing crystals. They helped me so much throughout my recovery and beyond.

Thanks to Louise, Sue and Claire for your angelic friendship along our journey of exploration. Special thanks also to Louise for your wonderful editing.

Thanks to Megs and Stuie for the read through and your much needed words of encouragement.

ACKNOWLEDGEMENTS

Thanks to Steven (a.k.a Polarbear) for having the balls to be heard and showing me it can be done.

Thanks to all the lovely nurses and Doctors at the NHS who kept me going.

Thanks to Kettley for your friendship, mentorship and complete understanding whilst I was ill.

Thanks to the amazing Owen crew for your love and understanding, Andy for your Big Bang visits, Judith for your editing eye and Pam for your prayers.

Last, but definitely not least – big up to the Rimells for your wonderful friendship! You guys never fail to make me laugh, and laughter is the cure to everything!

I hope that covers everyone. There are a few chunks of the journey that I still don't remember very well, so if I have forgotten anyone, please know that I am very grateful for your love and support.

Thank you. Thank you. Thank you. xxx

# ABOUT THE AUTHOR

**COMING SOON FROM CHARLOTTE JONES:**

**_To my BFF with CFS_**

A short eBook detailing the honest unfiltered advice Charlotte would give to her friends if they had CFS.

**_Cracks of Light_**

A book for everyone, sharing simple steps to bring light, joy, health and happiness into your life.

# ABOUT THE AUTHOR

Charlotte has been processing life through poetry since the age of five. Whilst experiencing extreme emotions, words repeat rhythmically in her head, over and over, until she gets them down on paper in the form of poetry. This inbuilt coping mechanism was a lifesaver throughout her time with CFS/ME/Fibromyalgia.

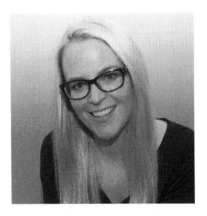

Having now made a full recovery, Charlotte lives a healthy, joyful, fulfilling life in England with her husband and son. She is grateful for all that she has learnt along her healing journey and now finds purpose in sharing this with others.

**To find out more about Charlotte's books and release dates, join her mailing list by visiting www.charlottejonesbooks.com**

Printed in the United States
By Bookmasters